Textbooks for the Four TCM Classical Courses

Selected Readings from *Shanghan Lun*

伤寒论选读

Compiler and Translator in Chief

Zhaozhi Cheng（成肇智）
Jiaxu Chen（陈家旭）

English Reviewer

Miguel Jose Rivero（Belize）

Contributors

Zhaozhi Cheng（成肇智）
Jiaxu Chen（陈家旭）
Douglas David Moore（Canada）
Miguel Jose Rivero（Belize）
Yanyun Liu（刘雁云）
Gangfeng Duan（段刚峰）
Xin Zhao（赵歆）
Yueyun Liu（刘玥芸）
Zhe Xue（薛哲）

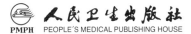

人民卫生出版社
PMPH PEOPLE'S MEDICAL PUBLISHING HOUSE

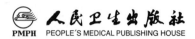

Website: http://www.pmph.com

Book Title: Selected Readings from *Shanghan Lun*
伤寒论选读（英文版）

Contact address: No. 19, Pan Jia Yuan Nan Li, Chaoyang District, Beijing 100021, P.R. China, phone: 8610 5978 7340, E-mail: zzg@pmph.com

First published: 2017
ISBN: 978-7-117-25554-7

ISBN 978-7-117-25554-7

Cataloguing in Publication Data:
A catalogue record for this book is available from the CIP-Database China.

Printed in The People's Republic of China

Acquisitions Editor: Rao Hongmei
Editor in Charge: Rao Hongmei
Book Design: Yin Yan   Bai Yaping   Shuichangliu

Look at the first published English textbooks of the TCM classics!

The Four Great TCM Classics are
  the **quintessence** of traditional Chinese medicine (TCM);
  the **fountainhead** of TCM academic theories;
  the **ladder** of TCM learners to success;
  the **source of expertise** for raising TCM physicians' clinical level;
  the **indispensable foundation** for TCM to spread toward the whole world.

Features of English Textbook of *Shanghan Lun*:

※ It was specially compiled & translated for TCM students, practitioners and the lovers of *Shanghan Lun* at home and abroad.

※ It contains 198 articles of original texts finely selected from *Shanghan Lun* and can reflect the diagnosis & treatment system on the basis of the six patterns and most important academic viewpoints in the classic.

※ There are 3 items for each article of the original text, i.e. synopsis, commentary and application, so it benefits much to comprehend the real meanings of the original texts and their clinical application.

※ By doing our best, the systematic English translations in this book has achieved its preciseness, conciseness and comprehensibility surely.

※ The textbook is suitable & convenient for teaching and self-learning, since it has been verified and revised from years of teaching experience, and distilled from lecture notes.

About Authors

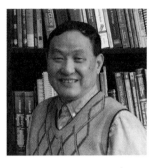

Prof. *Zhaozhi Cheng*, graduated from *Hubei* TCM University in China, and then worked at a countryside hospital in Western *Hubei* province as a TCM physician. Afterwards, he had taught *Neijing*, diagnostics and other courses in *Hubei* TCM University as an instructor, professor and mentor for doctoral candidate, and chiefly wrote and published 6 personal TCM works and 77 papers. Since 2007, he has been invited and come to Canada as a TCM senior instructor. Now he teaches four TCM classical courses, TCM internal medicine, Case Study and other TCM courses in both English and Chinese in PCU College of Holistic Medicine and *Tianyi* Health Group in Vancouver, and also engages in TCM clinical work as a registered TCM practitioner.

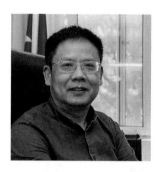

Dr. *Jiaxu Chen* is Chair Professor, *Changjiang* Scholar, Director of the State-Level Subject of Chinese Medicine Diagnostics in *Beijing* University of Chinese Medicine (BUCM). Chair Professor & Dean of School of Chinese Medicine, Jinan University (JNU), Director of TCM Formula-Syndrome Research Center of JNU, and Recipient of the Distinguished Young Scholar in National Science Foundation of China (NSFC).

He obtained his bachelor degree from *Hubei* University of Traditional Chinese Medicine in 1988, and further obtained his master's and Ph.D. degrees from BUCM. Dr. Chen is a specialist in traditional Chinese medicine. For many years, he has been concentrating his efforts on the research of traditional Chinese medicine, and has published more than 10 books and over 300 papers.

Being a renowned expert and academic in the field, Prof Chen has been appointed as Member of Committee of *Beijing* Natural Sciences Foundation, he also currently serves as Vice-Chairperson of Specialty Committee of Diagnostics of Traditional Chinese Medicine of World Federation of Chinese Medicine Societies (WFCMS), and Vice-Chairperson of Specialty Committee of *Li Shizhen* Medicine of WFCMS.

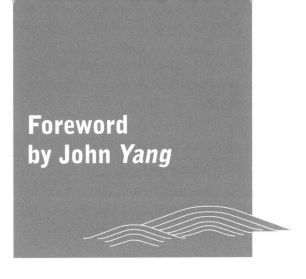

Foreword
by John *Yang*

In 2006, when I was the Dean and Clinic Director at the PCU College of Holistic Medicine, I had a difficult time finding a qualified faculty member to teach Traditional Chinese Medicine (TCM) in English. Not only was I looking for someone with a strong command of TCM knowledge, but also, someone who had the ability to teach classical TCM courses in English. In hopes of recruiting the perfect fit, my team ran a national advertising campaign, to which I found that none of the candidates met the necessary standards. My colleague then suggested that I begin to reach out to TCM universities in China. Again, unimpressed by the extremely small pool of eligible candidates, I searched until I found Professor *Zhaozhi Cheng* – a long-time PhD program mentor at the Hubei TCM University. Professor Cheng's accomplished 40-year teaching and research career did not go unnoticed; and I was eager to go through all the steps (including navigating the world of applying for special Canadian work visas) to ensure he would join the PCU team. Over the past 10 years, since his arrival to Canada and PCU College, Professor Cheng has solidified his reputation as an accomplished TCM practitioner, an excellent educator, and of course, a very popular classical TCM professor at the College.

As a highly respected TCM researcher and educator, I was delighted to learn that Professor Cheng was pursuing this important project. Readers: it may be your experience that English versions of TCM classics are devoid of comments from their respective authors, and are translated quite (too) literally. As you may know, the TCM classics were written in ancient Chinese. It is difficult for native Chinese speakers with classical TCM training to interpret, and even more so for those attempting to translate their original text from ancient Chinese into English. These TCM textbooks in English compile the specific excerpts from the TCM classics, and are masterfully structured in a way to help you foster a better understanding of original TCM paradigms. The most unique features of these books reflect in the "Commentary" and "Application" sections. I believe it was professor Cheng's intention to create both a theoretical and clinical text, and reflect the roots of acupuncture and Chinese herbal medicine. The sequence and manner of such originals were chosen both to present a culturally valid view of TCM and acupuncture, and to meet the needs of those who wish to study more sophisticated TCM theory and practice.

Suitable readers range from TCM students who wish to build a more solid foundation of TCM knowledge, and TCM practitioners hoping to find more success in their practices by learning subtle clues from the classics. Laymen seeking to learn basic principles of how to maintain health and wellness may also gain knowledge from reading these textbooks.

By John *Yang* Dr. TCM, PhD.

Dr. John *Yang* is a registered Doctor of TCM who resides in Vancouver, British Columbia, Canada. He earned his PhD in TCM from Guangzhou University of Chinese Medicine, and from 2003 to 2014, served as the Dean and Clinic Director at the PCU College of Holistic Medicine. Now he works at the *Kwantlen Polytechnic University*, the first public university in Canada to offer a TCM-Acupuncture program, as the program developer and department head. As an expert in the field, Dr. *Yang* has given many national and international presentations and lectures on TCM. He is the current President of the *Federation of Traditional Chinese Medicine Colleges of Canada* and a committee member on the *Standards Council of Canada, Canadian Advisory Committees for International Organization for Standardization for TCM*.

Foreword
by Joseph Ranallo

The *Huangdi Neijing, Shanghan Lun, Jingui Yaolue* and *Study on Warm Disease*, are known as the earliest and most important documents on the theoretical origin of Traditional Chinese Medicine (TCM). These texts guided the past human thinking away from the Daost shamanistic conviction that body disorders and diseases are caused by varied demonic pathogenic influences and refocused our thoughts on how our lifestyles and the universal forces impact our health and well being. This new approach stressed that our diet, emotions, and thinking, as well the varied laws, forces, energies, and universal postulates can and do affect our lives. These texts confirm that to sustain good health, we need to access and retain the balance level of these life and universal traits. The Classics contend that it is more important to prevent than to cure diseases. The best healing modalities, according to these texts, are those that can help us to meet these goals.

The *Huangdi Neijing* and other Classical texts claim that successful healing modalities feature these and other common components: Yin/Yang forces, the Five elements, health preservation, balanced mental states, the capacity to keep the body in balance as we age, and the safe and easy accessibility to effective treatments. Through analyzing symptoms and pulse, TCM practitioners can determine which viscera are becoming excessive or deficient. Because these imbalances can lead to diseases and other pathogens, practitioners can needle the appropriate acupoints or prescribe herbal formulas to rebalance the viscera, bypass the diseases, and, by so doing, maintain a health preservation status. The Classical TCM approach can provide patients with a healthy longevity. By keeping the Kidneys in balance, it can also assist patients to pass with ease through their childhood, adolescence, early adulthood, menopause/andropause, and senior phases. All of these life enhancements are prominently promoted by the TCM classics.

Along with a rapid spreading of TCM throughout the world, more and more foreign people, especially young persons, are studying and practicing TCM in China and at abroad now. I believe that the publishing of the textbooks of four TCM classical courses in English editions will not only fill up the blank space of the same kind of publications, but will also meet their demand for improvement of proficiency of both TCM theory and practice so as to make a greater contribution to the people's general health in the world.

By Joseph Ranallo BA, MA, R. AC.

Joseph Ranallo is a Registered Acupuncturist in British Columbia (B.C.), Canada. He holds a BA from the University of Victoria, and an MA from Washington State University. Joseph has taught and administered in schools at the Elementary, Secondary, College, and University levels. Since 2001, he has managed a part time Acupuncture Practice in Rossland, B.C. He has made academic presentations at major universities and events in Canada, U.S.A., Italy, and China. Joseph has taken an active role in the governance of his varied professions. In his TCM practice, he has served on the Board of ATCMA (B.C.'s largest Association of Traditional Chinese Medicine and Acupuncture Practitioners). Since 2016, he has been an elected member of the Board of Directors of CTCMA, the provincial regulatory body for Traditional Chinese Medicine.

Contents

Notes on Compilation and Translation   1

Brief Introduction to *Shanghan Lun*   4

Chapter I Differentiation of Symptoms, Pulses and Treatment of *Taiyang* Pattern

Section 1   **Outlines of *Taiyang* Pattern**   10
Article 1, 2, 3, 6, 4, 5, 7, 11

Section 2   ***Taiyang* Wind Invasion Syndrome**   18
2.1 **Principal syndrome and main formula**   18
Article 12, 13, 95, 24, 44, 15, 53, 54, 16, 17

2.2 **Concomitant syndromes of *Taiyang* wind invasion**   27
Article 14, 18, 43, 20, 62

Section 3   ***Taiyang* Cold Invasion Syndrome**   31
3.1 **Principal syndrome of *Taiyang* cold invasion**   31
Article 35, 36, 46, 47, 55

3.2 **Concomitant syndromes of *Taiyang* cold invasion**   36
Article 31, 32, 33, 38, 39, 40, 41

3.3 **Contraindications of excessive diaphoresis**   43
Article 83, 84, 85, 86, 87, 88, 89

Section 4   **Interior Syndromes of *Taiyang* Pattern**   45
Article 71, 74, 73, 106, 124, 125

Section 5   **Transmuted Syndromes of *Taiyang* Pattern**   53
5.1 **Diagnosing-treating key points of transmuted syndromes**   53
Article 16, 90, 91

5.2 **Heat syndromes transmuted from *Taiyang* pattern**   55
Article 76, 63, 26, 34

5.3 **Deficiency-cold syndromes transmuted from *Taiyang* pattern**   59
Article   64, 118, 112, 67, 102, 66, 61, 69, 82, 29, 177

5.4 **Chest-agglomeration syndromes**   72
Article   134, 135, 137, 138

5.5 **Epigastric stuffiness syndromes**   76
Article   151, 154, 155, 149, 157, 158

5.6 **Doubtful-similar syndromes of a transmuted one**   83
Article   161, 173, 159, 156, 28, 152, 166

5.7 ***Taiyang* syndromes with spontaneous relief**   91
Article   58, 59, 93, 94

Questions for Review and Thinking   92

Chapter   Ⅱ   **Differentiation of Symptoms, Pulses and Treatment of *Yangming* Pattern**

Section 1   **Outlines of *Yangming* Pattern**   95
Article   180, 182, 185, 183, 186, 181, 210, 211

Section 2   ***Yangming* Heat Syndromes**   99
Article   176, 219, 168, 169, 170, 228, 223

Section 3   ***Yangming* Obstruction Syndromes**   104
Article   248, 249, 207, 213, 214, 239, 215, 241,
255, 238, 220, 242, 212, 252, 253, 254, 247

Section 4   **Contraindication Syndromes for Purgation**   115
Article   204, 205, 206, 189, 194

Section 5   **Concomitant and Transmuted Syndromes of *Yangming* Pattern**   117
Article   236, 260, 199, 261, 262, 237, 257

Questions for Review and Thinking   122

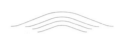

Chapter III Differentiation of Symptoms, Pulses and Treatment of *Shaoyang* Pattern

Section 1   **Outlines of *Shaoyang* Pattern**   125
Article 263, 97, 264, 265

Section 2   **Differentiation and Treatment of *Shaoyang* Pattern**   129
Article 96, 266, 101, 230, 229, 99, 100

Section 3   **Concomitant and Transmuted Syndromes of *Shaoyang* Pattern**   138
Article 267, 146, 103, 165, 147, 107, 172

Questions for Review and Thinking   145

Chapter IV Differentiation of Symptoms, Pulses and Treatment of *Taiyin* Pattern

Section 1   **Outlines of *Taiyin* Pattern**   147
Article 273, 277

Section 2   **Concomitant and Transmuted Syndromes of *Taiyin* Pattern**   149
Article 276, 163, 279, 280, 259

Questions for Review and Thinking   153

Chapter V Differentiation of Symptoms, Pulses and Treatment of *Shaoyin* Pattern

Section 1   **Outlines of *Shaoyin* Pattern**   155
Article 281, 282, 283, 285, 286

Section 2   ***Shaoyin* Cold-transformation Syndromes**   159
Article 323, 317, 315, 316, 304, 305, 307, 301, 302, 324, 372

Section 3   *Shaoyin* Heat-transformation Syndromes   170
             Article   303, 319, 320, 321, 322

Questions for Review and Thinking   174

Chapter   VI   Differentiation of Symptoms, Pulses and Treatment of *Jueyin*
               Pattern

Section 1   Major Syndrome of *Jueyin* Pattern   176
             Article   326, 338, 359

Section 2   Cold Syndromes of *Jueyin* Pattern   180
             Article   351, 352, 378, 309, 243

Section 3   Heat Syndromes of *Jueyin* Pattern   186
             Article   318, 371

Section 4   Differentiation and Treatment of Cold Limbs   189
             Article   337, 353, 335, 350, 355, 356

Section 5   Differentiation and Treatment of Vomiting and
             Diarrhea   192
             Article   377, 379, 370, 374, 373

Questions for Review and Thinking   194

Appendixes   List of Main Reference Books   195

             Index of Ordinal Number of the 198 Articles   196

             Index of the Formulas in this Book   198

Notes on Compilation and Translation

1. This book is for academic purposes, in other words, it is applicable to students studying traditional Chinese medicine (TCM) in English at home and abroad. Therefore, it can be used as a higher textbook for foreign students in Chinese universities or colleges of TCM, and also for students in TCM schools or colleges overseas. Furthermore, it is a popular book read for self-learning among the general public, who may themselves be experienced TCM practitioners for improving their clinical proficiencies, or those interested in TCM classics or the *Shanghan Lun*（伤寒论, *Treatise on Cold-Induced Disorders*）only.

2. TCM classics are archaic and complex in language, and diversified and profound in meaning, thus it is very difficult for today's people to understand all of its original text. For requirement and convenience of teaching, 198 articles and 74 formulas of the *Shanghan Lun*, which are seen as important and basic parts of the classic have been selected and compiled into this textbook, and are divided into six chapters, such as *Taiyang* pattern, *Yangming* pattern, *Shaoyang* pattern, *Taiyin* pattern, *Shaoyin* pattern and *Jueyin* pattern. Furthermore, each pattern is redivided into several sections according to their specific academic contents, such as their outline, principal syndromes, concomitant syndromes, transmuted syndromes and contraindicated syndromes.

3. In order to teach or self-studying the textbook conveniently and effectively, there are three items set up for each article, i.e., synopsis, commentary and application. Formerly, the original text of each article is expressed in black-thick scripts. The "synopsis" refers to a brief summary of the core idea of this article; the "commentary" refers to an analysis or explanation on the main academic viewpoints based on the "synopsis"; and finally, "application" points out the guiding significance of the article in both TCM basic theory

and clinical practice, or utilizes some examples to highlight its clinical application in the later ages. There are questions at end of every chapter in "for review and thinking" so as to direct students to precisely understand and firmly grasp the absolute learning content and major viewpoints in the chapter.

4. The classic concepts in *Shanghan Lun* selected and compiled into this text book, are based on the requirements for studying. The most originals in the book appear in identical chapters of the *Shanghan Lun*, with just a few articles as exceptions. The number of the articles are preserved in the book, but the article sequence has changed much in the light of teaching demand. Usually every article is dealt with alone, but sometimes two or more articles are dealt with together in one section due to their common ground in academic regard. In addition, some unnecessary or poorly understood topics of the original text in *Shanghan Lun* haven't been selected into this book.

5. The Chinese meanings of a part of characters and terminology in the original text have different explanations up to now, with only one meaning being generally acknowledged and adopted into this book, but a few words in the original text are explained in accordance with personal understandings of the compiler of this book. The purpose is minimizing perplexities arising among learners or readers when seeking an understanding of the material.

6. There are some characters, phrases and sentences in the original text of the *Shanghan Lun* that should be collated and then can be understood clearly and correctly. The most collated original text in this book are in accordance with the current text books in Chinese, however a few collations are presented through the compiler's comprehension.

7. It is very hard to accurately translate TCM writings from Chinese into English, especially when translating TCM classics, since there are no ready-made corresponding words, phrases and sentences in the English language. Consequently, this book is translated from Chinese into English by means of free translation methods, partly combined with word-for-word translation

and transliteration. Furthermore, the free translation is based on a combination of the corresponding Chinese character denotation and TCM theories.

8. Transliteration in this book is accompanied by Chinese phonetic alphabet in italics. Generally speaking, transliteration should be used as least as possible. Only a minority of the terms and phrases in this book are roughly translated into English, including some specialized TCM vocabulary that lack corresponding English expressions, and are translated using Chinese phonetic alphabet, such as *Yin-Yang*（阴阳）, *Qi*（气）, *Sanjiao*（三焦）, *Bianzheng Lunzhi*（辨证论治）, *Taiyang*（太阳）, names of persons, books, dynasties, meridians, Chinese herbal medicines, formulas and acupoints. Some TCM terms are translated with a combination of free translation and transliteration, e.g., *Zangfu*-organs（脏腑）, upper-*Jiao*（上焦）and so on.

9. When certain basic or important terms and phrases first appear, two translations with Chinese characters may be displayed simultaneously so as to easily comprehend the true meaning of these English expressions. Thereafter, one of the two is continuously used alone.

10. Some articles offer relevant prescriptions which are called classical formulas. Usually we introduce the ingredients and their doses of each formula as they first appear in the book; after that, only the name of the formulas are mentioned without their ingredients and doses. The dosages of Chinese medicines in each formula are commonly used clinically in the modern day, and not the original dosages of *Shanghan Lun*, during Eastern *Han* Dynasty for the sake of minimizing the readers' difficulty in dose conversion. By decreasing the length of the book, the methods of preparation and usage in only certain representative formulas are discussed, while others are omitted.

11. To facilitate study for the readers, indexes following the main reference books, ordinal number of the articles and the formulas used in this textbook are recorded at very end of the book.

Brief Introduction
to *Shanghan Lun*

1. Author, Writing Time and Its Rearrangement

Zhang Ji, also known as *Zhongjing,* lived in the later Eastern *Han* Dynasty (circa 150~219 AD), and is the greatest medical specialist in the history of TCM, and his main medical theories and clinical experiences were concentrated and embodied in his sole piece of academic work, namely, *Shanghan Zabing Lun* (Treatise on Cold-Induced and Miscellaneous Diseases) completed circa 200~205 AD, in which he established two medical theoretical systems, the six meridians pattern differentiation for exogenously contracted diseases and the syndrome differentiation according to theories of *Zangfu*-organs and *Qi,* blood and body fluid for miscellaneous diseases, and offered a vast number of formulas which have been effectively applied into clinical practice up to now. *Zhang*'s great work was rearranged into two books by an imperial medical officer, *Wang Shuhe* (210~285 AD), in the Western *Jin* Dynasty. One is *Shanghan Lun* (Treatise on Cold-induced Disorders) which mainly expounds the exogenously contracted diseases caused by wind-cold pathogen, and the other is *Jingui Yaolue* (Synopsis of the Prescriptions in *Golden Chamber*), which emphatically discusses miscellaneous diseases relating to TCM Internal Medicine, Surgery and Gynecology.

The current edition of *Shanghan Lun* was reorganized and collated by *Lin Yi* (circa 1065~1066 AD), who was head of official Bureau of Collating-Rectifying Medical Texts in the North *Song* Dynasty.

2. Basic Contents and Significance

The current edition of *Shanghan Lun* is divided into 10 chapters and 22 sections, containing 397 articles and 112 prescriptions. Among them, the major clinical manifestations, key points for differentiation, therapeutic rules and relevant formulas for basic patterns are the core contents. The important and most commonly used articles and formulas are selected and compiled into this teaching text book for the course.

The major contribution of *Shanghan Lun* to TCM can be expressed as the following three aspects:

① First setting up a complete diagnosing-treating system for exogenously contracted disease according to the six meridian patterns, entailing consistency of symptoms, pathogenesis, therapeutic rules and prescriptions.

② Formulation of very effective and concise prescriptions used for different patterns and syndromes, which have been known as classical formulas, and extensively applied not only in exogenously contracted diseases, but also in endogenously miscellaneous diseases.

③ Initiating a series of clinical thinking models which have guided TCM clinical work over 1800 years, especially in syndrome differentiation.

For this reason, this book has been considered as an ancestor to medical recipes, while *Zhang Ji* has been referred to as a medical sage.

3. Commonly used Terms in Differentiation of the Six Meridian Patterns

3.1 **Cold-induced disease**（*Shanghan* 伤寒）: In a narrow sense it refers to the exogenously contracted diseases mainly caused by cold or wind-cold pathogens; but in a general sense, it covers all exogenously contracted diseases caused by six exogenous pathogens and pestilential pathogens.

3.2 **Six meridian patterns**（*Liujing Bing* 六经病）: It contains the disorders of three *Yang* patterns, i.e., *Taiyang, Yangming* and *Shaoyang*, and disorders of three *Yin* patterns, i.e., *Taiyin, Shaoyin* and *Jueyin*. However, the six meridian patterns in *Shanghan Lun* don't only refer to the disorders of the twelve regular meridians, but should also be understood as the comprehensively pathological concepts, which refer to the six basic pathological patterns of exogenous diseases in different stages (early, middle and later stages), natures (cold or heat, excess or deficiency) and locations (exterior or interior, involveing the pathological layers from the superficial to the deepest and different *Zangfu*-organs respectively). Moreover, one of such six meridian patterns may be divided into more concrete syndromes.

3.3 Principal syndrome（*Zhuzheng* 主证）: The fundamental and representative syndrome among many syndromes of each pattern, usually treated by a basic formula, thus a principal syndrome can be named with its basic formula treating it.

3.4 Concomitant syndrome（*Jianzheng* 兼证）: A more complicated syndrome consisting of a principal syndrome and one or several symptoms differing in the pathogenesis of the principal syndrome, and each principal syndrome may have several concomitant syndromes.

3.5 Transmuted syndrome（*Bianzheng* 变证）: A syndrome transformed from a principal syndrome into another syndrome due to delayed or wrong treatment, and thus the principal syndrome has disappeared.

3.6 Deteriorated syndrome（*Huaizheng* 坏证）: A serious or dangerous transmuted syndrome often caused by wrong treatment, so it can be seen as a special transmuted syndrome with greater severity than the principal one.

3.7 Contraindicated syndrome（*Jinji Zheng* 禁忌证）: One or several syndromes prohibited for treatment with a basic formula, hence the syndromes would worsen or become dangerous if the formula is used for this syndrome.

3.8 Doubtful-similar syndrome（*Nisi Zheng* 疑似证）: A syndrome similar to the principal syndrome or a main transmuted syndrome in a part of symptoms but is quite different from it. So it may be easily confused with another similar syndrome in diagnosis.

3.9 Concurrent occurrence of two or three patterns（*Hebing* 合病）: Two or more patterns appearing simultaneously, initially in the cold-induced disease.

3.10 Amalgamation of two patterns（*Bingbing* 并病）: One pattern occurring first, followed by another pattern, then both existing simultaneously.

3.11 Affection of both patterns（*Lianggan* 两感）: Two exteriorly - interiorly related patterns occurring at the beginning of the cold- induced disease.

3.12 Direct attack（*Zhizhong* 直中）: Exogenous pathogen invading directly into one of three *Yin* patterns, namely, one of three *Yin* patterns appearing at the initial stage of the cold-induced disease.

3.13 Sequential transmission（*Xunjing Chuan* 循经传）: Conventional way of transmission by patterns in cold-induced diseases along with the routine sequence as mentioned in the *Neijing*, i.e. *Taiyang→Yangming →Shaoyang→ Taiyin→Shaoyin→Jueyin*.

3.14 Skip-over transmission（*Yuejing Chuan* 越经传）: An unconventional transmission of a pattern skipping over another pattern or more, in the cold-induced disease.

3.15 Transmission from *Yang* pattern into *Yin* one（*Yangbing Ru yin* 阳病入 阴）: One of three *Yang* patterns developing into one of three *Yin* patterns, usually suggesting aggravation of the disease.

3.16 Transmission from *Yin* pattern outward *Yang* one（*Yinbing Chu yang* 阴 病出阳）: One of three *Yin* patterns transmitting onto one of three *Yang* patterns, often showing alleviation of the disease.

3.17 Main formula（*Zhufang* 主方）: The most effective and commonly used prescription for a specific syndrome.

4. Requirements and Methods for Learning the Course

This course entails 80 hours of instruction. Throughout the course, students are expected to learn the following:

① Grasping the main clinical manifestations, pathogeneses, treatment rules and prescriptions of the six patterns and their principal syndromes as well as commonly seen concomitant syndromes.

② Grasping the key points for syndrome differentiation between two similar or easily confused syndromes.

③ Become familiar with the main ingredients, basic actions, chief indications and clinical applications of the commonly used formulas in the *Shanghan Lun* as well as *Zhang Zhongjing*'s medication expierences.

④ Familiarizing yourself with the thinking models in TCM diagnosing-treating activities established by *Zhang Zhongjing* and then applying them into your own clinical practice.

While learning TCM classics like *Shanghan Lun*, it is recommended to utilize the following methods:

① Correctly and clearly understand the intrinsic meanings of every word and sentence in the original text you will learn throughout the course, especially knowing the precise meaning of a word or a phrase from its context, and referring to other closely related articles.

② Know well the meaning behind the original sentence of each article by means of ancient logical inference, such as inferring a formula from the symptoms or pulse given, inferring the symptoms or pulse from a formula given, and inferring the pathogenesis from a formula given.

③ Make a contrast or comparison between two similar articles or formulas in order to find out their similarities and differences.

④ Studying the original text in the *Shanghan Lun* would relate closely with the actual problems in clinical practice so as to have a more accurate and realistic command of the theory, viewpoints and principles in this classical course.

Questions for Review and Thinking

1. What kind of medical book do you think of *Shanghan Lun* to be? What understand do you have about its position and significance in TCM?

2. What does "Six meridian patterns" in *Shanghan Lun* refer to? Please give a brief explanation for the essence of each pattern!

3. What are the basic meanings of principal syndrome, concomitant syndrome and transmuted syndrome? How do you understand the relationships among them to be?

Chapter I

Differentiation of Symptoms, Pulses and Treatment of *Taiyang* Pattern

— **Article 1** —

In *Taiyang* pattern there must be floating pulse, headache with stiff nape, and aversion to cold.

Synopsis

An outline for differentiation of *Taiyang* pattern.

Commentary

The term *Taiyang* pattern in *Shanghan Lun* refers to the most superficial layer of the human body facing the invasion by exogenous pathogen first, so *Taiyang* pattern among the six meridian patterns usually refers to the wind-cold exterior syndrome in the early stage of exogenously affected diseases.

Since exogenous invasion by wind-cold leads to an intense struggle between vital *Qi* and the exogenous pathogen in the body surface, *Qi*-blood going outward results in a floating pulse, *Qi*-blood stagnation in the *Taiyang* meridian brings about headache with stiff nape, and defensive *Qi* failing to warm the body surface, and invasion of exogenous pathogens on the exterior body result in the aversion to cold. Moreover, fever is not mentioned here, because aversion to cold is serious but fever is relatively slight and appears later in wind-cold exterior syndrome.

In general, this article has been thought of the differentiation program for *Taiyang* pattern, and all of *Taiyang* syndromes in *Shang han Lun* should have such three symptoms to a different extent.

Application

Although these three symptoms are the principal basis for diagnosis of *Taiyang* pattern clinically, however, they may have different concrete manifestations in different patients and are not typical in some cases. For example, the floating pulse is often combined with other pulses, such as tense, moderate, rapid, thready and wiry pulses; headache may be commonly seen, but a stiff nape only seen in a minority of cases; and aversion to cold probably varies in degree, such as aversion to wind, intolerance of cold or even cold-shivering.

Meanwhile, fever and aversion to cold often occur in combination, and the fever in *Taiyang* pattern is usually mild and appears a bit later. Of course, the patients suffering from *Taiyang* pattern may have the other symptoms, such as stuffy nose with running nose, aching all over, uncomfortable or itchy throat, cough, etc.

Article 2

The *Taiyang* pattern marked by fever, sweating, aversion to wind, and moderate pulse is known as wind invasion syndrome.

Synopsis	A guideline for differentiation of *Taiyang* wind invasion syndrome.
Commentary	*Taiyang* wind invasion syndrome is a principal syndrome of the *Taiyang* pattern mainly caused by the patient's body with deficiency of defensive *Qi* and simultaneous invation by an exogenous wind-cold pathogen leading to disharmony between nutritive *Qi* and defensive *Qi*. This is also called wind-cold exterior deficiency syndrome. Here "*Taiyang* pattern" signifies the basic pathogenesis and manifestations mentioned previously in Article 1. Furthermore, fever and aversion to wind indicate an exterior syndrome arising from the wind pathogen attacking the body surface, and spontaneous sweating suggests weak defensive *Qi* failing to secure nutritive *Qi* and thus resulting in excessive opening of sweat pores. The observed moderate pulse here means loosened and a little feeble, due to exterior deficiency. In regard to Article 1 and 2, *Taiyang* wind invasion syndrome must present spontaneous sweating, aversion to wind, low fever, headache, and a floating-moderate pulse, all resulting from disharmony between nutritive *Qi* and defensive *Qi* due to exogenous invasion of the wind pathogen into body surface where defensive *Qi* is deficient.
Application	This article points out an mixture type of excess with deficiency in the

exogenous disease, namely, wind-cold exterior deficiency syndrome, and its focus for syndrome differentiation on spontaneous sweating with aversion to wind. It also suggests that both constitutional deficiency and the affected wind pathogen together play a decisive role in the occurrence of exogenously contracted diseases.

Article 3

The *Taiyang* pattern marked by the presence or absence of fever, certain aversion to cold, body aches, vomiting and a tense pulse felt over *Cun*, *Guan* and *Chi* portions, is called cold invasion syndrome.

Synopsis

A guideline for differentiation of *Taiyang* cold invasion syndrome.

Commentary

Taiyang cold invasion syndrome is another principal syndrome of *Taiyang* pattern caused by the body with a sound defensive *Qi* invaded by exogenous cold pathogen leading to stagnation of both defensive *Qi* and nutritive *Qi* with a severer obstruction of the meridian *Qi* due to cold pathogen tightening the body surface inward, also called wind-cold exterior excess syndrome. Whether fever is present or not, or fever appearing early or late, depends on a strong or weak defensive *Qi* obstructed by the cold pathogen. Severe aversion to cold with no sweating originates from exogenous cold tightening the exterior, then closing the sweat pores and obstructing the outward flow of *Yang Qi*. Body aches result from stagnation of meridian *Qi* and contraction of tendons-vessels by the cold invasion, vomiting from an adverse ascending of stomach-*Qi* induced by the pathogen, and tense pulse indicates severe cold attacking the exterior. Connecting with Article 1, main presentations of *Taiyang* cold invasion syndrome include aversion to cold, fever, no sweating, headache, body aches and floating-tense pulse.

Application

Comparing *Taiyang* cold invasion syndrome with *Taiyang* wind invasion syndrome, the former is mainly caused by a sound defensive *Qi* struggling against cold pathogen, and then serious stagnation of *Qi*-blood in the meridian, thus manifested as absence of sweating, aversion to cold, fever, severe pain and floating-tense pulse; whereas, the latter by deficient defensive *Qi* against wind pathogen, resulting in disharmony between nutritive *Qi* and defensive *Qi*, manifested as spontaneous sweating, aversion to wind, milder fever, mild aches and floating-moderate pulse.

Comparison between the Two Principal Syndromes
of *Taiyang* pattern

Syndrome	*Taiyang* wind invasion syndrome	*Taiyang* cold invasion syndrome
Similarity	Pathogenic wind-cold invading the exterior body; dysfunction of nutritive *Qi* and defensive *Qi*	
Different pathogenesis	Weak defensive *Qi* and dicharging out of nutritive *Qi*; wind is first pathogen	Stagnation of nutritive *Qi* and defensive *Qi*; cold is first pathogen,
Different symptoms	Spontaneous sweating, aversion to wind, fever, milder aches, a floating and moderate pulse	No sweating, aversion to cold, fever or no fever, severer pain, a floating and tense pulse

Article 6

The *Taiyang* pattern characterized by fever, thirst and absence of aversion to cold, is known as warm disease. If there is a generalized scorching fever after inducing sweating, it is named wind-warmth, which manifests as floating pulse on the *Cun, Guan* and *Chi* portions, spontaneous sweating, heavy sensation of the body, sleepiness, coarse snoring sounds while respiration, and slurred speech. If the warm disease is treated with purgatives, there would be dysuria, eyeballs fixed upward, and both urination and stool incontinence. If the warm disease is treated by fire therapy, there would be slightly yellow skin, and paroxysmal convulsions like epileptic attacks, and a dark-lusterless complexion like being fumigated by smoking in the severe cases. The first mistreatment may protract the course of the disease, and the second mistreatment may lead to a quicker death.

Synopsis   A guideline of *Taiyang* warm disease and its deteriorated syndromes caused by different mistreatment.

Commentary   *Taiyang* warm disease is one type of *Taiyang* pattern caused by the wind-heat pathogen and mainly marked by higher fever without obvious aversion to cold, thirst, headache, and floating-rapid pulse. However, it also suggests that "cold-induced disease" in a broad sense in *Shanghan Lun* refers to all of exogenous febrile diseases, and should be treated by pungent-cool drugs to relieve this exterior syndrome.

Taiyang warm disease would worsen and then be transformed into various deteriorated syndromes due to different erroneous treatment. A wrong diaphoresis with pungent-warm drugs may lead to a deteriorated syndrome called "wind warm" due to intense internal heat damaging *Qi* and body fluid, and disturbing the mind, so manifesting as high fever, profuse sweating, heavy body sensation, lethargy, coarse snoring sounds, slurred speech and a floating-swift-forceful pulse. Wrong purgation may result in serious *Yin* exhaustion and stir up liver wind, thereby presenting as dysuria or anuria, eyeballs fixed upward and both urinary and stool incontinence. Fire therapy, including warm-needling, direct moxibustion and hot medicated compress, cannot be used for heat syndromes, otherwise it would bring about extreme heat inducing liver wind, urgent jaundice with slightly yellow skin, frequent convulsion-like attacks of epilepsy, and a dark-lusterless complexion like being fumigated by smoke. A patient is going to die if such therapeutic mistakes are continuously made twice.

Application

This article had a profound influenc on the theories of Warm disease in the later ages. According to the major books of warm disease in *Qing* Dynasty, pathogenesis, symptoms, developing direction and treatment in the early stage of the warm disease are quite different from those in the cold-induced disease in a narrow sense. For example, a warm disease in early stage marked by severe fever, slight aversion to cold, less sweating, headache, thirst, sore throat, thin-dry tongue coating and a floating-rapid pulse, should be treated with pungent-cool drugs to expel wind-heat pathogen instead of pungent-warm drugs that mainly induce sweating, and *Yinqiao San* (银翘散) is a suitable formula.

Moreover, it easily turns into an intense internal heat, and further damages *Yin* instead of weakening *Yang*, disturbs the mind, and stirs up liver wind, thus manifesting as high fever, lethargy or coma, convulsion, acute jaundice and other serious and dangerous symptoms in the extreme stage of the warm disease. It is therefore necessary to clear away heat to detoxify, nourishing *Yin,* opening clear orifices and extinguishing liver wind, which have become commonly used therapeutic principles in the management of warm disease.

Finally, this article also proves on the contrary that warm disease can't be treated by diaphoresis with pungent-warm drugs and fire therapy, however, purgation with bitter-cold drugs can be used for interior excess-heat syndrome instead of *Yin* deficiency syndrome in the warm disease.

Article 4

On the first day of cold-induced disease, the pathogen invades *Taiyang*. If the pulse is still floating, it suggests the disease hasn't transferred; if there is severe nausea with vomiting, or restlessness, and a rapid and hurried pulse, it indicates the disease has transferred from *Taiyang* pattern into another one.

Article 5

On the second or third day of cold-induced disease, if there are no symptoms and signs of *Yangming* or *Shaoyang* pattern, this indicates that *Taiyang* pattern hasn't transformed.

Synopsis

Judgment of a transference of cold-induced disease depends upon the appearance of basic corresponding symptoms and pulse instead of the days calculated in advance.

Commentary

Transferring sequence of exogenous cold-induced disease in *Shanghan Lun* originated from *Huangdi Neijing*, i.e., *Taiyang→Yangming→Shaoyang→Taiyin →Shaoyin→Jueyin* from the first day to the sixth day. However, *Zhang Zhongjing* thought the course of any disease doesn't limit within only one fixed way to transfer, and it depends on a lot of factors, so patients' disease courses are always variable and ever changing, and diagnosis of transference of pattern or syndrome must be based primarily on the presenting symptoms, and it may keep the previous pattern without any transference if the main symptoms and pulse remain unchanged.

For this reason, judging the transference of *Taiyang* pattern must be according first to the clinical manifestations on hand instead of the others. Here, severe nausea with vomiting or restlessness and a rapid-hurried pulse can be observed respectively as the representative symptoms of *Shaoyang* or *Yangming* pattern, indicating that the *Taiyang* pattern has transferred into *Shaoyang* or *Yangming* pattern. However, if such symptoms have not appeared, the transference should be excluded.

Application

The viewpoint that transference of a disease from one pattern into another pattern is diagnosed on the basis of whether the main symptoms of another pattern are present or not, fully embodies *Zhang Zhongjing*'s valuable spirit of seeing truth in facts, which can be thought of not only as a theoretic source of *Bianzheng Lunzhi*, but also being one to be followed in clinical practice by the TCM doctors in later ages.

Article 7

Disease characterized by fever with aversion to cold belongs to *Yang* pattern, while that by aversion to cold without fever to *Yin* one.

Synopsis

The key point for syndrome differentiation between *Yin* pattern and *Yang* pattern in the cold-induced disease.

Commentary

Patterns of *Taiyang*, *Yangming* and *Shaoyang* belong to *Yang* syndrome, characterized by different typess of fever, i.e., *Taiyang* by fever with aversion to cold, *Yangming* by high fever without aversion to cold, and *Shaoyang* by alternate fever and chills. However, patterns of *Taiyin*, *Shaoyin* and *Jueyin* belong to *Yin* syndrome, characterized by different degrees of aversion to cold without fever. This is then considered a generalized clinical feature between syndromes of *Yang* and *Yin* in the

Shanghan Lun.

Application

Taking fever as a key symptom for deciding whether the *Yang* pattern or the *Yin* one in *Shanghan Lun* has been guiding TCM practice, especially in differentiation between *Yang* and *Yin* natures of disease up to now. However, this is but a general law, as there are some exceptions clinically. For instance, there is no fever but only aversion to cold acutely at the beginning of *Taiyang* cold invasion syndrome, and there is fever without aversion to cold in *Shaoyin* heat-transformation syndrome.

——— Article 11 ———

When a patient feels a hot body and desires for more clothes, it indicates cold in the bone marrow with heat in the skin; while a patient has a cold body and no desire for more clothes, it means heat in the bone marrow with cold in the skin.

Synopsis

Identifying a true or false cold and heat syndrome by means of patient's desire for cold or heat.

Commentary

Fever and aversion to cold are the chief symptoms of heat and cold syndromes, and simultaneous aversion to cold and fever are thought of the first manifestation of exterior syndrome. However, fever or aversion to cold may occasionally be false presentations of the real cold or heat syndromes, especially in the course of exogenous diseases. Therefore, this article points out that the patient's desire can be seen as an important basis for differentiating between true heat and cold syndromes.

Generally speaking, patient's desire for warmth or cool usually is a key point for differentiating true cold or heat in the interior body according to *Huangdi Neijing*. Here, feeling "a hot body" or "a cold body" belong to false symptomatology of the exterior, and desire or no desire "for more clothes" belongs to true symptomatology of the interior. Meanwhile, cold or heat "in the skin" signifies a false cold or heat symptom externally, but cold or heat "in the bone marrow" signifies presence of true cold or heat syndrome internally.

Application   A patient's desire or aversion can accurately reflect the nature of disease, so it has been used as one of the principal basis for judgment of the true pathogenesis of the patient. For example, desire for warm drinks and putting more clothes on suggests a cold syndrome or *Yang* deficiency, while desire for cold drinks and further undressing indicate a heat syndrome or *Yin* deficiency; abdominal pain getting better with applied pressure signifies a deficiency syndrome, and while it worsens when pressure is applied denotes an excess one.

Section 2 *Taiyang* Wind Invasion Syndrome

2.1   Principal syndrome and main formula

Article 12

Taiyang **wind invasion syndrome featured by outward floating of** *Yang Qi* **manifested as fever, and inadequate** *Yin* **fluid as spontaneous sweating, marked by mild aversion to cold, chilly aversion to wind, superficial fever, stuffy nose with coares noise and retching, should be treated mainly with** *Guizhi Tang.*

Guizhi Tang   *Gaizhi* 9 g, *Baishao* 9 g, *Shengjiang* 9 g, *Dazao* 3 pieces, and *Zhi Gancao* 6 g.

Break the above ingredients into small pieces, decoct them with 1400 ml water over a mild fire to get 600 ml decoction, and then remove the dregs. Take 200 ml of the decoction first at a warm temperature. Drink approximately more than 200 ml of hot gruel to reinforce the action of the decoction, shortly after taking the first dose. Then warm the patient's body by covering with a blanket to make the body skin moist due to slight sweating, but don't excessive sweating massively since the disease will not be relieved in this way. Cease taking the rest of the decoction if the disease is relieved with adquate sweating after taking the first dose; take the second dose in the same way if he has no sweating; and take the third dose in half a day while decreasing the period between two doses taken if sweating is still absent. If disease is severe, this decoction can be taken continueously throughout the day and carefully observe the patient's situation. Take another one or two packages of the same herbal medicines if the main symptoms are not resolved after finishing the first package of the decoction.

The foods including uncooked and cold foods and drinks, sticky and slimy foods, meats, noodles, the five acrid flavorings (the five strong-smelling vegetables, i.e., garlic, Chinese chive, Chinese leek, coriander and oil rape), liquor, milk products, and foods with a foul odor and spoiled quality, are all contraindicated while taking *Guizhi Tang*.

Article 13

Taiyang exterior syndrome with headache, fever, sweating and aversion to wind, should be treated mainly by _Guizhi Tang_.

| Synopsis | The basic pathogenesis, basic manifestations and main formula of *Taiyang* wind invasion syndrome. |

| Commentary | The two articles introduce the major symptoms, pulse and formula of *Taiyang* wind invasion syndrome, which arises from disharmony between nutritive *Qi* and defensive *Qi* induced by invasion of wind-cold in the exterior, in other words, wind-cold exterior syndrome with exterior deficiency, so low fever, aversion to wind, spontaneous sweating and floating-moderate pulse are regarded as key points for syndrome-differentiation. Here, "mild", "chilly" and "superficial" are used to vividly describe the clinical features of the fever with aversion to wind, which differ from *Taiyang* cold invasion syndrome, wind-heat exterior syndrome and others. Its accompanied symptoms may include headache, body |

aches, stuffy nose with coarse noise, retching, etc.

Guizgi Tang is the first formula in *Shanghan Lun* and also a basic remedy for *Taiyang* wind invasion syndrome. Among the ingredients in this formula, *Guizhi* with *ShengJiang* expels wind-cold to strengthen defensive *Qi* by inducing sweating, *Baishao* with *Dazao* nourishes blood and astringes nutritive *Qi*, and *Shengjiang*, *Dazao* and *Zhi Gancao* together can replenish stomach-*Qi* and assist *Guizhi* and *Baishao* to harmonize nutritive *Qi* and defensive *Qi*. Therefore, it has an intelligent combination of ingredients, and thus has a very effective clinical action. The preparation and administration of *Guizhi Tang* are here recorded in detail, and should be highlighted by students, because they are a part of essential of *Zhongjing*'s clinical experience in medication and also a necessary precondition for obtaining a satisfactory therapeutic effect. Furthermore, the preparations and administrations of the other formulas in this textbook might be identical to those of *Guizhi Tang* in principle, and subsequently those of others in the textbook will be left beyond their peculiarities.

| **Application** | 1. These two articles tell us the key points for differentiating *Taiyang* wind invasion syndrome from the others and using *Guizhi Tang* clinically, so we may correctly apply this formula in the light of key points, namely disharmony between nutritive *Qi* and defensive *Qi* with wind pathogen invasion, mainly marked by spontaneous sweating, aversion to wind, low fever, headache, and floating-moderate pulse. |

2. It offers an outstanding example for preparation and administration of herbal medicine in order to achieve the best therapeutic effect, so the other herbal medicines can be prepared and administrated in the similar way.

3. *Guizhi Tang* has been respectfully known as the ancestor of all herbal prescriptions, because it is not only the first formula in *Shanghan Lun* and a main formula for *Taiyang* wind invasion syndrome, but also it and its modified formulas such as *Guizhi Jia Gegen Tang*, *Guizhi Jia Houpo Xingren Tang*, *Guizhi Jia Fuzi Tang*, *Xiao Jianzhong Tang*, *Guizhi Xinjia Tang*, *Guizhi Jia Longgu Muli Tang*, *Danggui Sini Tang* and *Huangqi Guizhi Wuwu Tang*, are extensively applied in the concomitant

syndromes of *Taiyang* wind invasion syndrome as well as the endogenously damaged diseases due mainly to deficiency of both *Qi* and blood or both *Yin* and *Yang*.

Article 95

Taiyang pattern with fever and sweating suggests the outward floating of defensive *Qi* and inadequacy of nutritive *Qi*, which consequently cause fever and sweating respectively, and can be treated by *Guizhi Tang* efficiently in order to expel wind-pathogen.

Synopsis	The basic pathogenesis and treatment of *Taiyang* wind invasion syndrome.
Commentary	*Taiyang* wind invasion syndrome treated appropriately with *Guizhi Tang* involves two pathogeneses. Intrinsically, disharmony between nutritive *Qi* and defensive *Qi*, in other words, defensive *Qi* is obstructed by wind-cold in the body surface, and manifested as fever with aversion to wind, simultaneously, nutritive *Qi* involving in blood and body fluid lets out excesively, such as much spontaneous sweating resulting from inability of weak defensive *Qi* to secure the exterior body. Extrinsically, exogenous wind invades into the exterior and opens sweat pores, and further weakens defensive *Qi*. Therefore, the intrinsic and extrinsic pathogenic factors in combination lead to the *Guizhi Tang* syndrome.
Application	This article obviously points out that disharmony between nutritive *Qi* and defensive *Qi* combined with wind-cold invasion is the basic pathogenesis of *Taiyang* wind invasion syndrome, and also the indication of *Guizhi Tang*. Both have guided the theoretical explanation and clinical application of this syndrome and formula.

Article 24

Taiyang **pattern treated initially by** *Guizhi Tang***, but the exterior syndrome is unrelieved and furthermore vexation occurs, needling** *Fengchi*（风池 **GB20**）**and** *Fengfu*（风府 **GV16**）**first, the patient may recover after given** *Guizhi Tang* **once again.**

Synopsis *Taiyang* wind invasion syndrome with a stronger pathogen should be treated by using a combination of acupuncture and herbal medicines.

Commentary *Guizhi Tang* applied for *Taiyang* wind invasion syndrome is appropriate, but the syndrome is not relieved and a new symptom, vexation, is added, because a stronger wind pathogen gives rise to an intense struggle between vital *Qi* and pathogen, so as to cause a severer obstruction in the meridian, hence presenting vexation as one of the results of this pathological situation. Therefore, first needle acupoints *Fengchi* (GB20) and *Fengfu* (GV16) to expel exogenous wind to unblock the meridian, then give *Guizhi Tang* to expel the residual wind-cold pathogen by inducing mild sweating and harmonizing nutritive *Qi* and defensive *Qi*, so the severe case of *Taiyang* wind invasion syndrome may then be relieved completely.

Application It is a typical modality for applying herbal medicine and acupuncture together, which then enhance the therapeutic action because it gives full play to the strong points of the two therapies in regulating-reinforcing *Qi*-blood and unblocking the relevant meridian and collaterals respectively.

Article 44

Taiyang **pattern with unrelieved exterior syndrome cannot be inappropriately treated by catharsis, and should be treated appropriately by** *Guizhi Tang* **to relieve exterior syndrome.**

Synopsis The lingering *Taiyang* exterior syndrome can be treated exclusively by mild diaphoresis, instead of catharsis.

Commentary	The principal syndrome of *Taiyang* pattern lasting for a long time should be treated by mild diaphoresis, namely, using *Guizhi Tang* to induce sweating mildly only if the exterior symptoms still exist regardless whether it has been treated wrongly or not. However, *Taiyang* exterior syndrome can't be treated by catharsis, because catharsis would lead to damage of *Qi* of the *Zanfu*-organs, especially *Qi* of the spleen-stomach, and further deeper invasion of the exogenous pathogen, which then brings about some transmuted or deteriorated syndromes. Consequently, purgation is contraindicated for *Taiyang* exterior syndrome.
Application	Any syndrome within the six meridian patterns has its own specific pathogenesis, symptoms, therapeutic rule and major formula. When the key symptoms of a syndrome remain unrelieved, this basically indicates that the syndrome does not change, so the corresponding therapeutic rule and the formula can be still used. Moreover, *Guizhi Tang* belongs to mild diaphoretics, so it can be used for a lingering wind-cold exterior syndrome, whereas *Taiyang* pattern is a contraindication to cathartics.

Article 15

The *Taiyang* pattern with upward rushing of *Qi* after inappropriate catharsis may be still treated by *Guizhi Tang* with the preparation and administration method mentioned previously. If there is no upward rushing of *Qi*, this formula can't be given.

Synopsis	*Taiyang* pattern with upward rushing of *Qi* after wrong catharsis can be treated still with *Guizhi Tang*.
Commentary	"Upward rushing of *Qi*" here refers to a pathological tendency that the patient's vital *Qi* still tends to expel the pathogen upward and outward although the *Taiyang* pattern has been treated wrongly by catharsis, manifesting as a subjective symptom, i.e., a feeling of *Qi* rushing upward from the epigastric region to the throat, in addition to the exterior syndrome, so *Guizhi Tang* can still be used with the same preparation and administration mentioned in Article 12 in order to support vital *Qi* to

expel the pathogen by following the pathological tendency. Of course, absence of the upward rushing of *Qi* suggests vital *Qi* has been damaged seriously and the exterior syndrome has been transformed into the other transmuted syndrome, so *Guizhi Tang* cannot be given again.

| Application | *Guizhi Tang* used for *Taiyang* pattern with a feeling of *Qi* rushing upward in the chest suggests that the patient has a pathological tendency of vital *Qi* to expel the pathogen upward and outward, and this is an example of a clinical application of the therapeutic principle, "guiding a matter along its course of development" (*Yin Shi Li Dao* 因势利导）. |

Article 53

A disease characterized by frequent spontaneous sweating, means that the nutritive *Qi* is unaffected, yet not harmonized with the dysfunctional defensive *Qi*. Since nutritive *Qi* circulates within the vessels and defensive *Qi* flows outside the vessels, both should become well coordinated, and the patient will recover, after another induction of sweating. In such case, *Guizhi Tang* is available.

Article 54

A patient suffering from frequently and lingeringly fever and spontaneous sweating, has no disorders of the *Zangfu*-organs, implying a dysfunction of defensive *Qi*, and can be relieved through diaphoresis, thus *Guizhi Tang* is available for this.

| Synopsis | The pathogenesis and treatment of endogenous disease marked by frequent spontaneous sweating and lingering fever. |

| Commentary | Here, "a disease" refers to an endogenously damaged disease which takes spontaneous sweating as a chief symptom. Here "no disorders of the *Zangfu*-organs" means interior syndromes have been excluded. The |

diseases in both articles are caused by disharmony between nutritive *Qi* and defensive *Qi*, so *Guizhi Tang* can be used for harmonizing both by mild diaphoresis. In this case, the root cause of the disharmony lies in dysfunctional or weak defensive *Qi* instead of nutritive *Qi*, namely, inability of weak defensive *Qi* to secure nutritive *Qi*, leads to undue outward discharge of nutritive *Qi*, thus presenting frequent spontaneous sweating or with a lingering fever sometimes due to abnormal opening-closing of the sweat pores.

In *Guizhi Tang*, *Guizhi*, *Shengjiang* and *Zhi Gancao* strengthen defensive *Qi* (*Yang Qi*) to preserve nutritive *Qi* (*Yin* fluid), *Baishao* and *Dazao* nourish *Yin*-blood and reduce sweating by astringing, so the formula can cure this disorder.

Application

This is an extensive application of *Guizhi Tang* in endogenous miscellaneous diseases. In addition to *Taiyang* wind invasion syndrome seen in exogenous disease, *Guizhi Tang* can be also used for disorders due to disharmony between nutritive *Qi* and defensive *Qi* in endogenous diseases, manifested as frequent spontaneous sweating, or/and lingering fever, aversion to wind, easily catching a cold, lassitude, shortness of breath, dizziness, pale complexion and tongue, and thready-weak pulse, which can be treated by *Guizhi Tang*. In case of more serious deficiency of defensive *Qi*, this formula may be combined with *Yu Pingfeng San*（玉屏风散）, and in case of more serious *Yang* deficiency with persistent cold sweating, intolerance of cold, and cold-pain in limbs and joints, it can be combined with *Zhi Fuzi* and *Baizhu*. It is not necessary for the patient to cover with a blanket and drink hot porridge when taking this decoction since he has sweated much already.

—— Article 16

Guizhi Tang is originally for releasing muscular symptoms. If the patient has a floating-tense pulse, fever with no sweating, it is contraindicated. A physician should keep in mind so as not to make this mistake.

Article 17

If a heavy drinker suffers from exterior syndrome, *Guizhi Tang* cannott be given, otherwise it may cause vomiting because the sweet-warm quality would be unbearable.

Synopsis	Two contraindications of *Guizhi Tang*.

Commentary

Guizhi Tang can expel wind to relieve the exterior syndrome mildly, through harmonizing both defensive *Qi* and nutritive *Qi*, also known as "releasing muscular symptoms". This differs from the action of *Mahuang Tang*, i.e., expel cold to relieve exterior syndrome by strongly inducing sweating, so *Guizhi Tang* is used exclusively for wind-cold exterior deficiency syndrome instead of wind-cold exterior excess one, marked by aversion to cold with fever, absence of sweating, and a floating-tense pulse.

Guizhi Tang is sweet in flavor and warm in nature, and a person indulging in excessive alcohol drinking usually contracts damp-heat accumulation in the middle *Jiao*. Therefore, a heavy drinker takes *Guizhi Tang* will suffer from nausea, vomiting and epigastric stuffiness resulting from worsening damp-heat pathogen in the middle *Jiao* and further causing adverse ascending of stomach-*Qi*.

Application

Although *Guizhi Tang* has an extensive clinical application, however it belongs to the category of sweet-warm and tonifying-astringing formulas, thus cannot be used to treat *Taiyang* cold invasion syndrome and other interior heat or damp-heat syndromes.

Article 14

Taiyang **pattern marked by stiff and painful nape and back, with abundant sweating and aversion to wind, should be treated mainly with** *Guizhi Jia Gegen Tang.*

Guizhi Jia Gegen Tang	Original *Guizhi Tang* plus *Gegen* 12 g.
Synopsis	Main symptoms and treatment of *Tiayang* wind invasion syndrome with obstruction of the meridian *Qi*.
Commentary	Obvious stiff and painful nape and back, usually indicate severe obstruction of meridian *Qi*, especially *Qi* of *Taiyang* Meridian, and then involving in contraction of tendons and muscles in this area. This article discusses one of concomitant syndromes of the *Taiyang* pattern, i.e., *Taiyang* wind invasion syndrome with obstruction of the meridian *Qi*. Thus *Guizhi Tang* is used for the principal syndrome, and *Gegen* in a large amount is used for stiff and painful nape and back due to its actions in both unblocking the meridian and relaxing tendons-muscles, and also assisting *Guizhi Tang* with expelling wind to relieve the exterior syndrome.
Application	*Guizhi Jia Gegen Tang* can be used clinically for different diseases regardless of an absent exterior syndrome, such as stiff neck, headache, neurosis, common cold, urticaria, measles with unsmooth eruptions, and hypertension if there is solely obstruction of the meridian by the wind pathogen.

Article 18

A patient suffering frequently from dyspnea in combination with *Taiyang* wind invasion syndrome, should be treated by *Guizhi Jia Houpo Xingren Tang*.

Guizhi Jia Houpo Xingren Tang	adding *Houpo* 6 g and *Xingren* 9 g into *Guizhi Tang*.

Article 43

Taiyang pattern treated with wrong purgation is marked by slight dyspnea and unrelieved exterior syndrome, and should be treated mainly by *Guizhi Jia Houpu Xingren Tang*

Synopsis	Main symptoms and treatment of *Taiyang* wind invasion syndrome with adverse ascending of lung-*Qi*.
Commentary	*Taiyang* wind invasion syndrome with dyspnea, meaning panting, may be caused by frequent attacks of cough or asthma, and then contracted with exogenous wind-cold pathogen, or suffering from invasion of wind-cold pathogen first and then adverse ascending of lung-*Qi* due to delayed or wrong treatment. Therefore, on one hand, use *Guizhi Tang* to relieve *Taiyang* wind invasion syndrome; on the other hand, add *Houpo* and *Xingren* to reduce dyspnea by decending lung-*Qi* and dissoving phlegm.
Application	*Guizhi Jia Houpo Xingren Tang* is indicated clinically for acute attacks of chronic bronchitis, children bronchitis and bronchial pneumonia, marked by dyspnea or/and cough with expectoration of white sputum, itchy throat, sweating, aversion to wind or cold, white tongue coating and a floating-moderate pulse. In case of lung-heat, add *Huangqin*, *Sangbaipi* and *Shigao*; and in case of deficiency of lung-*Qi*, add *Shashen*, *Wuweizi* and *Hezi*.

Article 20

Taiyang pattern after excessive diaphoresis, marked by incessant leaking sweats, aversion to wind, dysuria, slightly contracted limbs with stiff and painful joints, should be treated mainly by *Guizhi Jia Fuzi Tang*.

Guizhi Jia Fuzi Tang	adding prepared *Fuzi* 9 g and *Zhi Gancao* 3 g into *Guizhi Tang*.
Synopsis	The clinical manifestations and treatment of *Taiyang* wind invasion syndrome with *Yang* deficiency due to excesive diaphoresis.
Commentary	Sweating depends on *Yang Qi* steaming body fluid, which induces sweats discharging out from the pores. Here "incessant leaking sweats" means profuse and ceaseless sweating, will not only consume body fluid, but also deplete *Yang Qi*. *Taiyang* exterior syndrome should be treated by appropriate diaphoresis, however, excessive diaphoresis surely damages exterior *Yang*, including defensive *Qi*, interior *Yang* and body fluid, so it manifests mainly as incessant leaking sweats, aversion to wind, dysuria with difficult urination, and contracted limbs with inability of joints to move freely. However, consider *Yang* and *Yin*, which is more seriously damaged? It is mainly dependent on the patient's body constitution. Inferring the pathogenesis from the formula used and according to original *Taiyang* wind invasion syndrome, *Yang* deficiency is primary, deficiency of body fluid is secondary, and also accompanied with slight exterior syndrome. Thus other accompanied symptoms may have aversion to cold, cold limbs, pale complexion, listlessness, pale tongue with white-thin coating, and deep-thready-slow or floating-weak pulse.

In *Guizhi Jia Fuzi Tang*, prepared *Fuzi*, *Guizhi* and *Shengjiang* together invigorate *Yang* of both exterior and interior of the body to secure *Yin*, next promote urination by enhancing *Qi*-transformation, and reduce contraction of the limbs by warming meridians and tendons; meanwhile, *Baishao*, *Dazao* and *Zhi Gancao* nourish *Yin* fluid, stop sweating by astringing, and relax the tendons and muscles to make the joints moving freely.

| Application | This formula has been commonly used for *Bi* (痹) disease, heart disease due to *Yang* deficiency, common cold due to wind-cold invasion with *Yang* deficiency, and spontaneous sweating due to *Yang* deficiency. When treating *Bi* disease with it, add *Fangfeng, Qinjiao* and *Weilingxian* in case of a severer wind pathogen; add *ChuanWu, Mahuang* and *Qianghuo* in case of severer cold pathogen; add *Cangzhu, Yiyiren* and *Mugua* in case of severer damp pathogen; add *Huangqi, Danggui* and *Jixueteng* in case of deficiency of *Qi* and blood; and add *Sangjisheng, Huainiuxi* and *Xuduan* in case of deficiency of the liver-kidney. |

Article 62

Taiyang exterior syndrome after inappropriate diaphoresis, marked by generalized pain and deep-slow pulse, should be treated mainly by *Guizhi Jia Shaoyao, Shengjiang Renshen Xinjia Tang* (abbreviated as *Guizhi Xinja Tang*).

Guizhi Xinjia Tang	adding *Baishao* 3 g, *Shengjiang* 3 g and *Renshen* 9 g into *Guizhi Tang*.
Synopsis	The main manifestations and treatment of *Taiyang* wind invasion syndrome with severe deficiency of both *Qi* and blood.
Commentary	*Taiyang* exterior syndrome unresolved after diaphoresis suggests the diaphoresis is not appropriate. Moreover, generalized pain here indicates the exterior pathogen hasn't been expelled completely, and also means failure of the skin, muscles and tendons to be nourished because of insufficiency of *Qi* and blood due to excessive sweating. A deep-slow pulse here shows serious deficiency of both *Qi* and blood (or defensive *Qi* and nutritive *Qi*). In addition to the above two main symptoms, there may be other presentations due to deficiency of *Qi* and blood, such as dizziness, listlessness, tiredness, spontaneous sweating, palpitations, shortness of breath, aversion to cold, numb limbs, pale complexion and tongue, and a thready-weak pulse.

For this reason, increase dose of *Baishao* to replenish *Yin* blood, increase dose of *Shengjiang* to strengthen *Yang Qi*, and add *Renshen* to tonify both *Qi* and blood. Meanwhile, *Guizhi Tang* can harmonize both defensive *Qi* and nutritive *Qi*, and expel the residual pathogen in the exterior.

Application   *Guizhi Xinjia Tang* is applied effectively for the common cold with deficiency of *Qi* and blood, bodily pain after either delivery or heavy bleeding, and wind-cold-damp *Bi* disease with deficiency of both *Qi* and blood.

Section 3   *Taiyang* Cold Invasion Syndrome

3.1   Principal syndrome of *Taiyang* cold invasion

Article 35

***Taiyang* pattern marked by headache, fever, bodily pain, lower back pain, joint pain, aversion to cold, absence of sweating, and dyspnea, should be treated mainly by *Mahuang Tang*.**

Mahuang Tang   *Mahuang* 9 g, *Guizhi* 6 g, *Xingren* 12 g and *Zhi Gancao* 3 g.

First decoct *Mahuang* with water 1200 ml to reduce water by 400 ml, and then remove the foams on the top of the decoction. Next, put the other medicines into the decoction and boil them until getting about 300 ml of decoction, then remove the dregs. Take orally 100 ml of the warm decoction as the first dosage. Cover with bedc lothes to induce mild sweating and don't eat porridge. The recuperation method of the patient is same as that of taking *Guizhi Tang*.

Synopsis   The basic manifestations and prescription of *Taiyang* cold invasion syndrome.

Commentary This article should be learned in combination with Article 3. *Taiyang* cold invasion syndrome is mainly caused by exogenous cold pathogen tightening the body surface, obstructing the meridian-*Qi* and blocking lung-*Qi*. Its basic manifestations are aversion to cold, fever (at the beginning there may be no fever), no sweating, headache with stiff nape, aching all over, dyspnea or cough, stuffy nose, and floating-tense pulse.

In *Mahuang Tang*, *Mahuang* expels wind-cold by inducing sweating and relieves dyspnea by dispersing lung-*Qi* outward and downward as the principal drug; *Guizhi* helps *Mahuang* in enhancing diaphoresis to expel wind-cold pathogen and unblocking meridian to reduce pain; *Xingren* assists *Mahuang* in dispersing lung-*Qi* outward and downward to reduce dyspnea and cough; and *Zhi Gancao* harmonizes all drugs, restrains excessive diaphoresis and reinforces vital *Qi*.

Application *Mahuang Tang* syndrome is obviously different from *Guizhi Tang* syndrome. Pathologically, its leading pathogen is cold instead of wind, the patient's defensive *Qi* is strong instead of weak, and stagnation of *Qi*-blood in meridian is more serious, so it is also called wind-cold exterior excess syndrome without deficiency. Symptomatically, absence of sweating, severer aversion to cold with fever, serious pain in the whole body, dyspnea with cough, and a floating-tense pulse are its clinical features, and are also seen as the fundamental basis for applying *Mahuang Tang*.

Clinically, this formula possesses multiple actions, such as inducing sweating, relieving pain, stopping dyspnea or asthma, promoting urination, anti-allergy and so on. Therefore, it is extensively used for common cold, influenza, chronic bronchitis, bronchial asthma, measles with pneumonia, allergic rhinitis, urticaria, nephritis with edema, facial paralysis, and rheumatic arthritis, which are all caused by wind-cold invasion into the exterior and the lung, followed by blockage of lung-*Qi*.

Comparison between the Syndromes of
Guizhi Tang and Mahuang Tang

Syndrome		*Guizhi Tang* Syndrome	*Mahuang Tang* Syndrome
Similarity		both belong to *Taiyang* pattern caused by exogenous wind-cold invading in the exterior body	
Difference	**Pathogenesis**	Exogenous wind invasion in the exterior with weak defensive *Qi* and letting out nutritive *Qi*, pertaining to wind-cold exterior deficiency syndrome.	Exogenous cold invasion in the exterior with stagnation of defensive *Qi* and nutritive *Qi*, pertaining to wind-cold exterior excess syndrome.
	Main Symptoms	Spontaneous sweating, aversion to wind, headache, fever, floating and moderate pulse.	No sweating, aversion to cold, severe headache and body pain, fever or fever, floating and tight pulse.
	Concomitant Syndrome	Deficiency of both *Qi* and blood, or disharmony of defensive *Qi* and nutritive *Qi*, leading to endogenous fever, spontaneous sweats.	Adverse ascent of the lung *Qi*, marked by acute exogenous cough and dyspnea.
	Therapeutic Principle	Expelling wind to ease muscles; and harmonizing nutritive *Qi* and defensive *Qi*.	Inducing sweating with pungent-warm to relieve exterior syndrome and dispersing lung *Qi*

Article 36

Concurrent occurrence of *Taiyang* and *Yangming* patterns characterized mainly with dyspnea and chest fullness, can not be treated by catharsis, for which *Mahuang Tang* is suitable.

Synopsis   Concurrent occurrence of *Taiyang* and *Yangming* patterns marked by more serious *Taiyang* cold-invasion syndrome can be treated adequately by *Mahuang Tang*.

Commentary   This article discusses a complex syndrome of *Taiyang* pattern and *Yangming* pattern occurring simultaneously, but the pathological emphasis must be placed on the *Taiyang* cold invasion syndrome, because its chief symptoms are dyspnea and chest fullness, which are attributable to blockage of the lung-*Qi* due to exogenous tightening by wind-cold, so its main pathological location is the exterior and the lung (*Taiyang*) instead of the stomach and large intestine (*Yangming*). Moreover, according to the basic principle of treatment in *Shanghan Lun*, while the exterior and interior syndromes appearing simultaneously, usually treating the exterior syndrome first and then treating the interior one, if the latter is not urgent or serious. Therefore, *Mahuang Tang* should be used for this syndrome first, and then treat the milder *Yangming* syndrome, or both syndromes may also be relieved after sweating. Catharsis is a basic therapeutic rule for *Yangming* obstruction syndrome caused by heat and dry stool together obstruction in the large intestine. If catharsis is used first for this complex syndrome, it would worsen because of deep invasion of the exterior pathogen and damage of spleen-stomach.

Application

This is a flexible usage of *Mahuang Tang* for the complex syndrome but *Taiyang* cold invasion syndrome is first indication. Meanwhile, the formula can also be used for cold-excess syndrome of asthma or cough, but without obvious exterior syndrome.

—— Article 46 ——

Taiyang pattern marked by a floating-tense pulse, no sweating, fever, and bodily pain, but unrelieved after lasting for 8 or 9 days, indicates the exterior symptoms are still present, so it should be treated by *Mahuang Tang* to induce sweating. If the condition slightly improves after taking it, and moreover the patient gets vexed and reluctant to open his eyes due to photophobia, or even nosebleed in the severe cases, and such symptoms can be relieved after nosebleed, because of heavy stagnation of *Yang-Qi* by the pathogen.

—— Article 47 ——

Taiyang pattern marked with a floating-tense pulse, fever and no sweating, may be relieved through automatic nosebleed.

Article 55

Taiyang cold invasion syndrome with a floating-tense pulse, but lack of diaphoresis in time leading to nosebleed, should be treated by _Mahuang Tang_ mainly.

Synopsis

Concentrated discussion on main symptoms and treatment of a severe _Taiyang_ cold invasion syndrome as well as relationship between taking _Mahuang Tang_ and nosebleed.

Commentary

Taiyang cold invasion syndrome hasn't been relieved for 8 or 9 days, which indicates the wind-cold pathogen and the patient's _Yang Qi_ are both strong, thus there is a heavy obstruction of _Yang Qi_ by the pathogen, and the use of _Mahuang Tang_ is too weak for this case, leading to vexation and reluctance to open the eyes with photophobia, along with a little improvement after taking the medicine. Since the patient has heavy _Yang Qi_ stagnation by the pathogen, and the exterior syndrome with residual pathogen can be expelled through nosebleed, which shows a sound ability of self-adjusting and self-controlling capability in the body, then the syndrome would be completely relieved finally.

However, _Taiyang_ cold invasion syndrome in some cases may be relieved automatically after nosebleed, or the syndrome with nosebleed but without inducing sweating can be still treated by _Mahuang Tang,_ because taking the decoction and occurrence of nosebleed share some common mechanisms, i.e., dispersing _Qi_, blood and body fluid to relieve exterior syndrome and diminish stagnated or excessive _Yang-Qi._

Application

The pathogen in exterior-excess syndrome can be dispersed outward by inducing sweating or nosebleed. In this case, nosebleed has a samilar action of expelling pathogen outward like inducing sweating; for this reason, it has been known as "red sweat" by some medical ancestors in the past. It must be pointed out that such therapies are only used for exterior-excess syndrome, in which abundant _Yang Qi_ is heavily obstructed by exogenous pathogen. Clinically, blood-letting from superficial collaterals commonly used for the exterior-excess syndrome and excess-heat syndromes, can be thought of a creative application of the viewpoint of "red sweat".

3.2   Concomitant syndromes of *Taiyang* cold invasion

─────── **Article 31** ───────

Taiyang pattern with a stiff and painful nape and back, no sweating and aversion to cold, should be treated mainly by *Gegen Tang*.

Gegen Tang	*Gegen* 12 g, *Mahuang* 9 g, *Guizhi* 6 g, *Baishao* 6 g, *Shengjiang* 9 g, *Dazao* 3 pieces and *Zhi Gancao* 6 g.

─────── **Article 32** ───────

Concurrent occurrence of *Taiyang* and *Yangming* syndromes often accompanied with spontaneous diarrhea should be treated mainly by *Gegen Tang*.

Synopsis	The symptoms and treatment of *Taiyang* cold invasion syndrome with stagnation of the meridian *Qi* or clear *Yang* sinking.
Commentary	*Taiyang* pattern with no sweating and aversion to cold implies a *Taiyang* cold invasion syndrome or wind-cold exterior-excess syndrome treated by *Mahuang Tang*. Here, stiff and painful nape and back signifies a severe obstruction in the *Taiyang* meridian, so should be treated by *Gegen Tang*, in which *Mahuang, Guizhi* and *Shengjiang* together relieve the exterior-excess syndrome by drastic diaphoresis, *Baishao, Dazao* and *ZhiGancao* nourish *Yin*-blood, prevent excesive sweating and also reduce the stiff pain by relax the tendons and muscles, moreover, *Gegen* in a larger dose can expel wind to relieve exterior syndrome, and unblock the meridian-*Qi* to relieve the stiff pain on the nape and back.

Article 32 discusses a complex syndrome of *Taiyang* and *Yangming,* in which *Taiyang* exterior-excess syndrome is first, and *Yangming* pattern marked mainly by a spontaneous diarrhea, caused by sinking of clear *Yang* instead of a wrong treatment, therefore, *Guizhi Tang* plus *Mahuang* is used for the former, and *Gegen* for the latter by its lifting the clear *Yang* to relieve diarrhea.

Application	*Gegen Tang* can be seen as *Guizhi Tang* plus *Gegen* and *Mahuang*, thus it has a strong action in inducing sweating to relieve exterior syndrome, unblocking meridian to reduce pain, lifting clear *Yang* to stop diarrhea and promoting eruption outward. At present, the formula has been applied extensively for common cold, influenza, chronic bronchitis, early stage of pneumonia, allergic rhinitis, nasosinusitis, conjunctivitis, facial paralysis, trigeminal neuritis, otitis media, periarthritis, cervical spondynosis, rheumatism in neck, sciatic neuritis, chronic colitis, acute gastroenteritis, measles, chicken pox, and allergic dermatitis.

Article 33

Concurrent occurrence of *Taiyang* and *Yangming* syndromes with vomiting but no diarrhea should be treated mainly by *Gegen Jia Banxia Tang*.

Gegen Jia Banxia Tang	Add *Banxia* 12 g into *Gegen Tang*.
Synopsis	Treatment of *Taiyang* and *Yangming* complex syndrome with vomiting.
Commentary	The syndrome discussed in this article is basically same as that in Article 32, the difference lies in either diarrhea or vomiting. The former is marked by vomiting instead of diarrhea, suggesting *Taiyang* cold invasion syndrome with an obstruction of meridian *Qi* and adverse ascending of stomach-*Qi*, but without sinking of clear *Yang*, so *Banxia is* added into *Gegen Tang* for descending stomach-*Qi* to stop vomiting.
Application	*Banxia* used for vomiting by descending turbid *Qi* and *Gegen* used for diarrhea by lifting clear *Qi*, fully demonstrate *Zhang*'s clinical experience

and feature in medication, which is one of the emphases that the TCM practitioners learn from *Shanghan Lun*.

Article 38

Taiyang exterior syndrome with a floating-tense pulse, fever, aversion to cold, bodily pain, absence of sweating, and fidgets, should be treated mainly by *Da Qinglong Tang*. It cannot be taken in case of faint or weak pulse, or even much sweating with aversion to wind, otherwise there will be cold limbs, twitching tendons and flesh, thus indicating a wrong treatment.

Da Qinglong Tang	*Mahuang* 18 g, *Guizhi* 6 g, *Xingren* 9 g, *Zhi Gancao* 6 g, *Shigao* 30 g, *Shengjiang* 9 g and *Dazao* 3 pieces.

Article 39

Taiyang cold invasion syndrome with a floating-moderate pulse, no pain but heaviness in the body, alleviated sometimes, with no symptoms of *Shaoyin* pattern, may be treated by *Da Qinglong Tang* to induce sweating.

Synopsis	The typical and atypical clinical manifestations and treatment of *Taiyang* cold invasion syndrome with interior heat, and contraindication for use of *Da Qinglong Tang*.
Commentary	*Taiyang* exterior syndrome marked mainly with fever, aversion to cold, absence of sweating, bodily pain and a floating-tense pulse, but fidgets probably combined with thirst and polypnea denote interior heat in the lung, which maybe caused by the patient's constitutional *Yang*-excess plus obstruction of defensive *Qi* due to exogenous wind-cold invasion, so here no sweating and fidgets are both key points for exterior-cold excess syndrome with interior heat, and thus should be treated by *Da Qinglong Tang*.

Da Qinglong Tang is *Mahuang Tang* with doubling the dose of *Mahuang*, decreasing dose of *Xingren*, and adding *Shigao, Shengjiang* and *Dazao*, thus it has a very strong action to induce sweating and also clear away internal heat. That is why it cannot be used for exterior-deficiency syndrome or *Yang* deficiency syndrome marked by spontaneous sweating, aversion to wind and faint or weak pulse, and it can't be used repeatedly or for prolonged period, otherwise, it may lead to depletion of *Yang* due to massive sweating.

However, the syndrome treated by *Da Qinglong Tang* in Article 39 is not so typical, because of varying kinds and severity of pathogens, and different types of body constitution, manifested as bodily heaviness without pain, with some symptoms fluctuating spontaneously, a floating-moderate pulse, no *Shaoyin* symptoms except aversion to cold, all of them can be seen as a severe damp and fluid-retention in the exterior with internal heat pathogen.

Application

Da Qinglong Tang has been used now for infection of the upper respiratory tract, influenza, bronchitis, pneumonia, epidemic meningitis, measles, acute arthritis, bronchial asthma, acute nephritis, erysipelas and so on, only if it is caused by exterior cold excess syndrome with interior heat. Generally speaking, *Mahuang* in a larger amount and *Guizhi* are used in case of more serious exterior cold, while *Shigao* is used in a larger amount or plus *Huangqin, Sangbaipi* and *Zhizi* in case of more serious interior heat. Besides, this formula shoulde be used cautiously because of its strongest diaphorestic action.

Article 40

Taiyang cold invasion syndrome with unrelieved exterior syndrome and fluid-retention in the chest and epigastric region, marked by retching, fever, cough, and possibly thirst, or diarrhea, or difficult swallowing feeling in the esophagus, or dysuria with fullness in the lower abdomen, or dyspnea, should be treated mainly by Xiao Qinglong Tang.

| *Xiao Qinglong Tang* | *Mahuang* 9 g, *Guizhi* 9 g, *Baishao* 9 g, *Banxia* 12 g, *Xixin* 9 g, *Ganjiang* 9 g, *Zhi Gancao* 9 g and *Wuweizi* 9 g. |

| **Synopsis** | The pathogenesis, clinical presentations and treatment of *Taiyang* cold invasion syndrome with fluid-retention. |

| **Commentary** | This is another concomitant syndrome of *Taiyang* cold invasion syndrome. "*Taiyang* cold invasion syndrome with unrelieved exterior syndrome" refers to aversion to cold, fever, no sweating, headache, bodily pain and a floating-tense pulse still present. Meanwhile, there is another pathogenesis "fluid-retention in the chest and epigastric region", where the fluid-retention staying in the stomach and esophagus gives rise to retching, thirst but no desire for drinking or desire for warm drinks, and difficult swallowing feeling in the esophagus; then attacking the lung upward to cause cough and dyspnea, flowing downward into the intestines to cause diarrhea with borborygmus, and retaining in the urinary bladder to cause dysuria with fullness in the lower abdomen. |

Xiao Qinglong Tang is actually *Mahuang Tang* minus *Xingren* and plus *Ganjiang, Xixin, Banxia, Wuweizi* and *Baishao,* in which, *Mahuang, Guizhi* and *Xixin* together expel wind-cold to relieve exterior syndrome by diaphoresis and also dissipate fluid-retention by promoting urination; *Ganjiang, Banxia, Xixin* and *Guizhi* can warm the lung to dissolve fluid-retention and then relieve cough and dyspnea; and *Baishao, Wuweizi* and *Zhi Gancao* support *Qi* and *Yin* and avoid undue warming-dispersing effect of the others by their tonifying-astringing action. Therefore, it has two basic functions: one is warming *Yang* to remove fluid-retention in the lung and stomach, another is relieving exterior cold syndrome by mild diaphoresis, and is thus suitable for cold fluid-retention in the lung with a mild exterior-cold syndrome.

| **Application** | *Xiao Qinglong Tang* right now has been applied extensively for acute and chronic bronchitis, bronchial asthma, senile emphysema, pneumonia, whooping cough and so on, as long as they share the pathogenesis of cold fluid-retention in the lung no matter whether there is exterior cold syndrome or not. The main symptoms and signs for applying this formula are cough, asthma or dyspnea with expectoration of profuse white, clear |

and thin sputum or foam-like sputum, aggravated in cold weather, alleviated in warm weather, stuffy or suffocative chest, or inability to lie flat, aversion to cold, especially on the back, pale complexion, pale-puffy tongue with white-slippery coating, and wiry-tense pulse. Increase the dose of *Ganjiang* in case of newly affected patients, increase the dose of *Wuweizi* in case of prolonged ones, remove *Mahuang* and *Xixin* in case of exterior-deficiency syndrome. It is not suitable for cough and dyspnea due to *Qi* or *Yin* deficiency syndrome although it is clinically safe.

Article 41

Taiyang **cold invasion syndrome with fluid-retention in the chest and epigastric region is marked by cough, mild dyspnea, fever, no thirst, should be treated mainly by** *Xiao Qinglong Tang***. When the patient feels thirsty after taking the decoction, it means that the cold fluid-retention is going to be disssolved.**

Synopsis

A further discussion on the basic pathogenesis, symptoms and treatment of *Taiyang* cold invasion syndrome with fluid-retention, and the evidence that *Xiao Qinglong Tang*has made a curative effect.

Commentary

This article stresses that cough and dyspnea are the key symptoms of *Xiao Qinglong Tang* syndrome because its chief pathogenesis is fluid-retention in the lung. "Fever" here suggests exterior syndrome, while "no thirst" arises from fluid-retention in the stomach.

If the patient feels thirsty after taking *Xiao Qinglong Tang*, it indicates that cold fluid-retention has been disssolved after taking the decoction. In this case, thirst is not severe and can be relieved automatically after drinking a little water. However, there possibly may be thirsty when the fluid-retention pathogen in the stomach obstructs the normal distribution of body fluid into the mouth, which should then be trerated with *Xiao Qinglong Tang* to dissolve fluid-retention by warming *Yang* as mentioned in the last article.

Da Qinglong Tang and *Xiao Qinglong Tang* are both used for the concurrent exterior and interior syndromes, but the former has a strong action to induce sweating and clearing heat, so is used for severe exterior cold syndrome with interior heat, while the latter has a strong action to warm *Yang* and dissolve fluid-retention in the lung and stomach, so is used for severe cold fluid-retention in the chest and epigastrium with mild exterior cold syndrome. Thirst occurring before or after taking a formula can be seen as one sign for judging the curative effect of a formula and prognosis of a patient over time.

Comparison between Two Syndromes of *Da Qinglong Tang* and *Xiao Qinglong Tang*

Syndrome		*Da Qinglong Tang* Syndrome	*Xiao Qinglong Tang* Syndrome
Similarity		Both concomitant syndrome of *Tayang* cold invasion; simultaneous appearance of exterior and interior sydromes	
Difference	Pathogenesis	*Taiyang* wind-cold exterior excess severer than lung-heat	Cold fluid-retention in lung with mild wind-cold exterior
	Actions of the formula	Strong diaphoresis with mild clearing away lung-heat	Strongly warm lung to dissolve fluid-retention with mild diaphoresis
	Key-points for differentiation	Severe aversion to cold, fever, no sweating, headache and body pain, vexation and dry mouth, reddish tongue with white coating, floating-tense-rapid pulse	Severe cough and dispnea, expectoration of profuse, thin or foamy sputum, suffocative chest, intolerance of cold, pale-puffy tongue with white-slippery coating and tense-wiry pulse

3.3 Contraindications of excessive diaphoresis

Article 83

A patient with dry throat can not be treated by diaphoresis.

Article 84

A patient suffering frequently from stranguria can't be treated by diaphoresis, otherwise hematuria may occur.

Article 85

A patient suffering frequently from sores-carbuncles with bodily pain cannot be treated by diaphoresis, because convulsion may occur after sweating.

Article 86

A patient suffering frequently from nosebleed can not be treated by diaphoresis, and spasmodic vessels sunken on the temples, staring forward with fixed eyeballs and inability to fall asleep may be observed after sweating.

Article 87

A patient suffering frequently from various types of bleeding cannot be treated by diaphoresis, otherwise aversion to cold with shivering may occur.

Article 88

A patient suffering frequently from profuse sweating cannot be treated by diaphoresis, otherwise distraction and lethargy with palpitations and pain in the genitals after urination may occur due to sweating inappropriately twice.

Article 89

A patient with cold pathogen in the interior cannot be treated by diaphoresis, otherwise cold-deficiency in the stomach may lead to vomiting out roundworms may occur.

Synopsis

principal contraindications to drastic diaphoresis with pungent-warm medicines.

Commentary

Sweating results from *Yang Qi* steaming body fluid in the exterior body, so appropriate diaphoresis can expel the pathogens out from the exterior body. However, wrong usage of inducing sweating may cause some harmful results clinically. For instance, diaphoresis cannot be used for the patients with dry throat, interior cold, or frequently suffering from stranguria, sores-carbuncles, nasal bleeding, hemorrhagic disorders and excessive sweating, because they have an underlying deficiency of *Yin, Yang, Qi* and blood, or have intense heat or damp-heat in the interior, thus improper diaphoresis would easily deteriorate their current diseased situations, then more serious and dangerous disorders marked by exaustion of vital *Qi* and rampant pathogens may occur, manifested as convulsion, cold-shivering, distraction, hemorrhage, or even depletion of *Yin* or *Yang* of the body leading to death.

Application	The contraindications for drastic diaphoresis therapy with pungent-warm medicines in *Shanghan Lun* are suitable not only in exogenously affected diseases, but also in endogenous miscellaneous diseases. Furthermore, they have been observed by TCM doctors over a long time.

Section 4   Interior Syndromes of *Taiyang* Pattern

——— Article 71 ———

After *Taiyang* pattern has been treated with diaphoresis, there is a lack of body fluid in the stomach due to excessive sweating, marked by fidgets, insomnia and desire to drink water, a small amount of water may be given and then the patient will recover due to normalization of the stomach. If a floating pulse, scanty urine, slight fever and thirst with unceasing drinking occur, *Wu Ling San* should be used primarily.

Wu Ling San	*Zexie* 15 g, *Fuling* 9 g, *Zhuling* 9 g, *Baizhu* 9 g and *Guizhi* 6 g
Synopsis	Differentiation of the thirst in *Taiyang* pattern after inducing sweating, and the main symptoms and treatment of water-retention syndrome in the bladder.
Commentary	This article basically discusses the formation, main manifestations and treatment of *Taiyang* water-retention syndrome in which body fluid is retained in the urinary bladder due to disturbance of *Qi*-transformation. Unduly inducing sweating leads to a lack of body fluid in the stomach, thus manifesting as desire to drink water, fidgets and insomnia due to both mild interior heat arising from relative deficiency of body fluid in the upper *Jiao*

and middle *Jiao*, and the heat transformed from exterior pathogen, so it can be relieved by giving a small amount of water. However, if drinking too much water beyond capacity of the kidney and spleen in *Qi*-transformation, then this leads to pathogenic water retention in the lower *Jiao*, manifested as dysuria, distending pain in the lower abdomen, slight fever, fidgets, insomnia, thirst with drinking and a floating-rapid pulse, which are caused by lack of body fluid in the upper body arousing internal heat, and the exterior syndrome still exists partially.

In *Wu Ling San*, *Zexie*, *Zhuling* and *Fuling* together remove Water retention by inducing diuresis, *Baizhu* and *Guizhi* warm *Yang* of spleen-kidney to promote *Qi*-transformation and then indirectly inducing urination; meanwhile, and *Guizhi* also expels residual exterior pathogen to relieve exterior syndrome. Therefore, it is suitable for *Taiyang* water-retention syndrome（*Taiyang Xushui Zheng* 太阳蓄水证）.

| Application | *Wu Ling San* has been applied not only for *Taiyang* water-retention syndrome in *Shanghan Lun*, but also for *Huoluan*（霍乱）with severe vomiting and diarrhea, fluid-retention with cough and dyspnea, edema, dysuria-anuresis, hernia and jaundice as long as they are all attributed to water or fluid retention in the body due to disturbance of *Qi*-transformation. It can be used extensively to treat acute and chronic nephritis, enteritis, infectious hepatitis, ascites due to cirrohsis, urinary infection, retention of urine, anuria, retention of gastric juice, Meniere's disease, cranial edema, glaucoma, diabetes insipidus, etc.. When applying it clinically, decoction taken warmly instead of powder taken with boil water is more common, and the dose of *Zexie* should be increased as usual. |

Article 74

When *Taiyang* wind invasion syndrome with fever is not relieved after six or seven days, both exterior and interior syndromes remain present, marked by desire to drink water but immediately vomiting while ingesting it, which is known as water counter-flow（*Shuini* 水逆）, for which *Wu Ling San* is used as the primary formula.

| Synopsis | The clinical manifestations and treatment of severe water-retention syndrome. |

| Commentary | This article expounds a syndrome called "water counter-flow", which can be seen as a severer type of *Taiyang* water-retention syndrome, and mainly caused by adverse ascending of stomach-*Qi* arising from an upward attack by water pathogen from the lower *Jiao* into middle *Jiao*. In addition to the basic clinical manifestations in Article 71, there is a chief symptom, i.e., desire to drink water but immediately vomiting while ingesting water. Since the pathogenesis of this disorder is similar to that in Article 71, *Wu Ling San* is the formula of choice. |

| Application | Clinically, *Wu Ling San* is often applied for disorders due to water or fluid-retention in the lower or middle *Jiao* no matter whether there is coexistence of exterior syndrome or not. This formula is originally a kind of powder taken with rice-cooked water, however, it has been used as a decoction in over the ages. |

Article 73

The cold-induced disorder with sweating and thirst, should be treated mainly by *Wu Ling San*; if without thirst, treated by *Fuling Gancao Tang*.

| *Fuling Gancao Tang* | *Fuling* 6 g, *Guizhi* 6 g, *Shengjiang* 9 g and *Zhi Gancao* 3 g |

| Synopsis | Differetiation and treatment of the syndromes of water retention in the lower *Jiao* and middle *Jiao*. |

| Commentary | The first paragraph still discusses *Taiyang* water-retention syndrome, sweating suggests a relieved exterior syndrome after diaphoresis, and thirst here must accompany with dysuria, distention-fullness in the lower abdomen and fidgets, so should be treated by *Wu Ling San*.

The second paragraph emphasizes the symptom, no thirst, implying the water pathogen in the middle *jiao*, especially in the stomach, thus |

accompanied with naursea, vomiting, epigastric stuffiness, poor appetite and cold limbs, since adverse ascending of stomach-*Qi* and *Yang Qi* obstructed by water retention.

Fuling Gancao Tang is *Ling Gui Zhu Gan Tang* minus *Baizhu* and plus *Shengjiang*, so it stronger than *Wu Ling San* in warming the stomach to dissolve water, but weaker in promoting urination by enhancing *Qi*-transformation.

<table>
<tr><td>Application</td><td>Comparing with *Ling Gui Zhu Gan Tang*, *Fuling Gancao Tang* is stronger in warming the stomach to dissolve water and lowering *Qi* to relieve vomiting. Thus this formula is used for disorders similar to *Ling Gui Zhu Gan Tang*, however, its clinical indication scope is narrower, often used to treat nausea, vomiting, epigastric stuffiness and splashing sound.</td></tr>
</table>

Article 106

Taiyang pattern is unrelieved and then the pathogenic heat and blood stasis agglomerate in the lower abdomen, manifested as mental disorders like mania, and possibly resolving spontaneously if the stagnated blood could be discharged from the anus. It should be treated by relieving exterior syndrome first, instead of purgation to remove blood stasis when the exterior syndrome is still present. If the exterior syndrome has been relieved and there is only tension-hardness or pain in the lateral lower abdomen, purgatives can be used, and *Taohe Chengqi Tang* is appropriate in this case.

<table>
<tr><td>Taohe Chengqi Tang</td><td>*Taoren* 12 g, *Dahuang* 12 g, *Guizhi* 6 g, *Mangxiao* 6 g and *Zhi Gancao* 6 g.</td></tr>
<tr><td>Synopsis</td><td>The primary symptoms and treatment of mild *Taiyang* blood-retention syndrome, and the principle of first relieving exterior syndrome if associated with it.</td></tr>
<tr><td>Commentary</td><td>Unrelieved *Taiyang* pattern may be transformed into pathogenic heat and blood stasis agglomerating in the lower abdomen because of the exterior pathogen converted into internal heat and then combined with blood</td></tr>
</table>

stasis, which may be latent in the small intestine or result from blood concentrated by the heat pathogen; this is called as *Taiyang* blood-retention syndrome (*Taiyang Xuxue Zheng* 太阳蓄血证) in later ages. There are obvious symptoms as tension-hardness or pain in the lateral lower abdomen with tenderness, mental disorders like amnesia and mania, and hematochezia like tar, which arise from blood stasis combined with heat staying in the lower *Jiao*, disturbing mind and enforcing blood extravastion. The other clinical presentations may be fever, headache, thirst, vexation, normal urination, and a deep-forceful-rapid pulse.

In *Taohe Chengqi Tang*, *Taoren* and *Guizhi* promote blood circulation to remove stasis, *Dahuang* and *Mangxiao* clear heat and eliminate blood stasis by purgation, and *Gancao* protects stomach-*Qi* and diminishes drastic action of the others, so it is appropriate for this syndrome.

Application

Traditionally, *Taohe Chengqi Tang* has been used extensively for blood stasis and heat agglomeration in any part of the human body not only in the lower *Jiao*, and its modifications have been already applied for acute pelvic inflammation, chronic pyelonephritis in the oliguric stage of epidemic hemorrhagic fever, excess-heat type of apoplexy, vascular headache, adhesive ileus, schizophrenia, allergic purpura, hemoptysis in the lung tuberculosis, postpartum hematoma, postpartum mania, persistent flow of lochia, retention of separated placenta, dysmenorrhea, premenstrual headache, traumatic hematoma, fracture of lumbar vertebra, chronic and appendicitis, only if they are all caused by blood stasis and blood heat in combination.

Article 124

After *Taiyang* pattern that lasts for six or seven days, exterior syndrome still exists, with a slightly deep pulse, no chest-agglomeration symptoms, and mania suggesting blood stasis with heat retention in the lower *Jiao*, full-hard lateral and lower abdomen, and normal urination, it should be treated mainly with *Didang Tang* to discharge the stagnated blood from the anus. This is because both blood stasis and heat pathogen together in the interior result from deeper invasion of the pathogen along the *Taiyang* meridian.

Didang Tang	*Shuizhi* 9 g, *Mangchong* 9 g, *Zhi Dahuang* 9 g and *Taoren* 6 g
Synopsis	The clinical presentations, pathogenesis and treatment of severe *Taiyang* blood-retention syndrome.
Commentary	The *Taiyang* exterior syndrome lasting for six or seven days shows the pathogen and vital *Qi* both are strong, and a slightly deep pulse suggests *Taiyang* pathogen has invaded into the interior, absence of chest-agglomeration syndrome excluding phlegm-water and heat combined in the upper *Jiao* and middle *jiao*; however, mania, fullness-hardness in the lower abdomen, normal urination and recovery after discharge of blood stasis out, all signify *Taiyang* pathogen has invaded from the exterior into the interior along the meridian, and then blood stasis and heat pathogen agglomerating in the lower *Jiao*.
	Since mania, full-hard abdomen and a deep-unsmooth pulse are more serious than those in *Taohe Chengqi Tang* syndrome, it is called severe *Taiyang* blood-retention syndrome, and should be treated by *Didang Tang*, which has a stronger action to remove blood stasis and a weaker action to clear heat by purgation because of *Shuizhi* and *Mangchong* in this formula and no *Mangxiao* in it.
Application	We must be cautious when using *Didang Tang,* which has a very strong action to remove blood stasis and probably arouses some severe bleeding and other toxic reactions, so we should be extremely cautious to use it for pregnant women, old patients and debilitated people, and it can't be used for prolonged periods.
	Now the formula can be used for abdominal masses, amenorrhea, external injuries, hepatosplenomegaly in the late stage of schistosomiasis, and tubercular peritonitis, likely due to serious blood stasis.

**Comparison beteen *Taiyang* Water-Retention and
Blood-Retention Syndromes**

	Syndrome Name	*Taiyan* water- retention syndrome	*Taiyang* blood- retention syndrome
Similarity		*Taiyang* pathogen from the exterior into the interior *Fu*-orgen; presenting fullness-distention in the lower abdomen and fever.	
Difference	Pathogenesis	Water-retention in the bladder due to *Yang* deficiency leading to disturbance of *Qi*-transformation with mild exterior syndrome.	The heat pathogen coming from the exterior into the *Fu*-organ combined with blood stasis in the lower *Jiao*.
	Main manifestation	Dysuria, distention in the lower abdomen, thirst with desire for drinks, or vomiting, fidgets, floating-rapid pulse	Smooth urination, contracted, stabbing pain with tenderness, mania, purplish or ecchymosed tongue, deep-knotted pulse.
	Treatment	Warming *Yang* to enhance *Qi*-transformation, inducing urination to expel water.	Eleminating blood stasis to unblock meridian, clearing heat by purgation.

—— Article 125

Taiyang **pattern marked by yellowish skin, deep-knotted pulse, hardness in lateral-lower abdomen and oliguria, which indicate absence of blood stasis. When urination is smooth and insanity like mania occurs, it shows a definite blood-retention syndrome, and should be treated mainly by** *Didang Tang.*

Synopsis

A supplement to the symptoms and pulse of *Taiyang* blood-retention syndrome and the key points for differentiation between damp-heat jaundice and blood-retention syndrome.

Commentary

This article first mentions two symptoms, namely, yellowish skin and deep-knotted pulse. However, yellowish skin with deep-knotted pulse may result from either blood stasis in the lower *Jiao* or damp-heat retention in the liver and spleen leading to jaundice disease, the former is accompanied with hardness-fullness or stabing pain in lateral-lower abdomen, insanity like mania, dark-lusterless complexion or sallow skin, smooth flow of urination, and hematochezia; but the latter with abdominal distention, oliguria or dysuria, jaundice with bright yellow color like orange peel, vexation but no manic symptoms, nausea, vomiting, disgust at food, red tongue with yellow-greasy coating, etc.. Meanwhile, deep-knotted pulse here suggests a severe interior excess syndrome and a deep stagnation of *Qi*-blood.

Application

Both *Didang Tang* and *Taohe Chengqi Tang* can be used for syndrome of blood stasis with interior heat, but the former is used for severer blood stasis with mild heat, while the latter for severer heat and obvious intestinal obstruction with milder blood stasis.

This article also suggests yellow skin may be caused by severe blood stasis with interior heat, so some types of *Yang* jaundice can be treated by removing blood stasis and clearing heat to cool blood.

In addition, *Didang Tang* can be prepared from decoction into pill for chronic or mild cases of *Taiyang* blood-retention syndrome.

Contrast between Two *Taiyang* Blood-Retention Syndromes

Syndrome	*Taohe Chengqi Tang* Syndrome	*Didang Tang* Syndrome
Pathogenesis	Milder blood stasis and severer interior heat with intestinal obstruction	Severer blood stasis and milder interior heat
Main Symotoms	Contraction and distention in the lower and lateral abdomen, mental disorder like mania, fever, thirst, reddish-dark tongue with yellow-dry coating.	Hardness and fullness in the lower and lateral abdomen with tenderness, mania, alleviation after discharging out of blood stasis, purplish or ecchymosed tongue and deep-knotted pulse.
Therapeutic principle	Clearing away heat to cool blood and removing blood stasis by purgation after relieving exterior syndrome.	Strongly eliminating blood stasis to unblock meridian first, next mildly clearing away heat.

Section 5   Transmuted Syndromes of *Taiyang* Pattern

5.1   Diagnosing-treating key points of transmuted syndromes

Article 16

***Taiyang* pattern lasting for three days that hasn't been relieved after inducing diaphoresis, emesis, purgation or warm needling, may become a deteriorated syndrome, thus *Guizhi Tang* cannot be given. Carefully inspect the patient's pulse and symptoms, know what new pathogenesis entails, then treat it according to present clinical manifestations.**

Synopsis	Concept of deteriorated syndrome and basic therapeutic principle for transmuted syndrome caused by mistreatment of *Taiyang* pattern.
Commentary	A deteriorated syndrome is a special type of the transmuted syndromes because it is severer than other transmuted syndromes, and due to mistreatment of the principal syndrome, such as wrong diaphoresis, emesis, purgation and warm needling.
	Next, the basic therapeutic principle of transmuted syndrome is aming at its pathogenesis, which is evidenced with the patient's symptoms and pulse.
Application	In the *Shanghan Lun* a transmuted syndrome means the principal syndrome transformed into a new one in which the pathogenesis differs from that of original one, therefore, its treatment is also completely different. This is also a theoretical source of *Bianzheng Lunzhi*, i.e., the most important principle of diagnosis and treatment in TCM.

Article 90

It is wrongful to use purgation for a disorder which should originally be treated by inducing sweating; while it is not wrong if inducing sweating is used first. It is also wrong for diaphoresis to be adopted for a disorder for which purgation should be original treatment; hence, it is not wrong if purgation is applied first.

Article 91

Cold-induced disease after being mistreated by purgation presents incessant diarrhea with undigested food in stool and bodily pain, should be treated urgently by relieving the interior syndrome, so *Sini Tang is* suitable. After that, defecation becomes normal and there is still bodily pain, then *Guizhi Tang* should be used timely to relieve the exterior syndrome.

Si Ni Tang	raw *Fuzi* 15 g, *Ganjiang* 9 g and *Zhi Gancao* 6 g
Synopsis	The priority of treatment for concurrent exterior and interior syndromes.
Commentary	In the progressive course of exogenous disease the exterior syndrome and interior syndrome may appear simultaneously, so a priority of treatment given to the exterior syndrome or interior one should be considered carefully. There are three basic principles to deal with such complicated situations, e.g., relieving exterior syndrome first by *Guizhi Tang* for diaphoresis if interior one is not serious or urgent; secondly, treating the interior syndrome urgently by *Sini Tang* to restore *Yang Qi* to save the life or by purgatives to preserve *Yin* fluid first when interior syndrome is serious or urgent; thirdly, treating the exterior syndrome and interior one at the same time while both are equally serious.
Application	The therapeutic principles in these two articles can be seen as concrete and flexible application of *Biao-Ben* treatment in the *Neijing*, and have influenced deeply the TCM clinical practices for a long time.

Article 76

Severe vomiting after inducing sweating suggests inappropriate diaphoresis, and the second diaphoresis will lead to ceaseless vomiting and diarrhea. A patient has vexation, inability to fall asleep, tossing about in bed and extreme distress in severe cases after such diaphoresis, emesis and purgation; this should be mainly treated by *Zhizi Chi Tang*. If it is associated with shortness of breath, *Zhizi Gancao Chi Tang* should be used. If it is associated with vomiting, *Zhizi Shengjiang Chi Tang* should be used.

Zhizi Chi Tang	*Zhizi* 9 g and *Dandouchi* 30 g.
Zhizi Gancao Chi Tang	add *Zhi Gancao* 6 g into *Zhizi Chi Tang*.
Zhizi Shengjiang Chi Tang	add *Shengjiang* 15 g into *Zhizi Chi Tang*.
Synopsis	Differentiation and treatment of vexation with insomnia due to heat disturbing around the chest and diaphragm.
Commentary	*Taiyang* pattern has disappeared after wrong treatment, and the heat pathogen that had transformed from exterior pathogen, then deeply invades into the chest and diaphragm, then disturbs mind, and is marked by some symptoms arising from a restless mind, such as vexation, inability to fall asleep with tossing about in bed, and extreme distress. The other symptoms include suffocation in chest, hot feeling in the heart, bitter taste and dryness in the mouth, red tip of tongue with thin-yellowish coating, and a floating-rapid pulse. All of the manifestations indicate heat pathogen in the *Qi* phase of the upper *Jiao* disturbing the mind and obstructing *Qi* flow in the chest.
	In *Zhizi Chi Tang, Zhizi* clears away heat from the chest and diaphragm to calm mind, and *Dandouchi* disperses stagnated heat outward to diminish

vexation and suffocation, both together are very suitable for this syndrome. Add *Zhi Gancao* to strengthen *Qi* in case of shortness of breath; then add *Shengjiang* to lower stomach-*Qi* in case of vomiting.

<table>
<tr><td>Application</td><td>*Zhizi Chi Tang* has been used in the later ages as a basic formula for vexation, insomnia, distress in cheat, low fever, and dry mouth pertaining to mild cases of heat pathogen in the *Qi* phase of upper *Jiao*, no matter if it comes exogenously or endogenously.</td></tr>
</table>

Therefore, it is effectively applied to treat such diseases as dysfunction of autonomous nerves, neurosis, gastritis, hepatitis and viral myocarditis at present, and usually combined with dispersing wind-heat drugs, such as *Chaihu, Bohe* and *Jinyinhua*, clearing heat drugs as *Huanglian, Zhuye* and *Lianqiao*, nourishing *yin* drugs as *Baihe, Shengdihuang* and *Maidong*, and dissipating phlegm drugs as *Zhuru, Beimu* and *Gualou*.

——— Article 63 ———

After inducing sweating, *Guizhi Tang* cannot be used again. If there are sweating, dyspnea and no high fever, it can be treated with *Mahuang Xingren Gancao Shigao Tang*.

<table>
<tr><td>*Ma Xing Shi Gan Tang*</td><td>*Shigao* 30 g, *Mahuang* 9 g, *Xingren* 9 g and *Zhi Gancao* 6 g.</td></tr>
<tr><td>Synopsis</td><td>The clinical manifestations and treatment of dyspnea resulting from heat pathogen being congested in the lung after diaphoresis.</td></tr>
<tr><td>Commentary</td><td>*Taiyang* pattern treated by inappropriate induction of sweating, will result in excessive sweating, dyspnea and still fever which indicate the exterior pathogen transformed into heat that invades the lung, leading to an adverse ascending of lung-*Qi,* marked chiefly by dyspnea. Here, "sweating" means no *Taiyang* exterior syndrome is present, so "*Guizhi Tang* cannot be used", and "no high fever" suggests lack of *Yangming* heat syndrome but intense heat pathogen obstructing the lung-*Qi*. The other symptoms of this</td></tr>
</table>

syndrome may have stuffy chest, cough with a little yellow-thick and stticky sputum, or even the inability to lie flat, thirst, restlessness, red tip or edge of tongue with a yellow-dry coating, and slippery-rapid or floating pulse.

Ma Xing Gan Shi Tang has a strong action to clear lung-heat and disperse lung-*Qi* outward and downward to relieve dyspnea, for which *Shigao* with *Mahuang* clears away lung-heat, *Xingren* helps *Mahuang* descending lung-*Qi* to reduce dyspnea, and *Gancao* harmonizes all drugs and also dissipates phlegm to normalize the lung.

Application

Ma Xing Gan Shi Tang has been commonly used as a basic formula for cough and dyspnea due to intense lung-heat with less phlegm and whether exterior syndrome is present or not, also it is extensively applied in the treatment of common cold, influenza, bronchitis, bronchial pneumonia, bronchial asthma, measles complicated with pneumonia, whooping cough, acute pharyngitis and laryngitis. In this case, *Shigao* should have a large dose, and the ratio between Mahuang and Gancao is 5:1. This formula cannot be used for cold type and deficiency type of diseases with dyspnea or/and cough.

Article 26

When a patient sweats profusely after taking *Guizhi Tang*, marked by heavy fidgets and thirst, even though drinking much water and surging-large pulse, *Baihu Jia Renshen Tang* is used as a main formula.

Baihu Jia Renshen Tang

Shigao 50 g, *Zhimu* 18 g, *Jingmi* 30 g, *Gancao* 6 g and *Renshen* 10 g.

Synopsis

The primary manifestations and treatment of *Yangming* heat syndrome with obvious impairment of body fluid and *Qi* due to inappropriate use of *Guizhi Tang*.

Commentary

Taiyang pattern treated by *Guizhi Tang* has been converted into an intense interior heat syndrome, marked with high fever, profuse sweating, heavy fidgets and thirst, drinking large amount of water and surging-rapid pulse, which indicate the heat pathogen has transformed from the exterior syndrome of *Taiyang* pattern, deeply invaded into *Yangming,* and *Yangming* heat syndrome with obvious deficiency of both body fluid and *Qi,* thus *Baihu Jia Renshen Tang* can be used to clear away heat in *Qi* phase and complement *Qi* and body fluid. Actually, this is an example for transformation of *Taiyang* pattern into *Yangming* one, which belongs to intense excess-heat with deficiency of *Qi* and *Yin.* In this formula, *Shigao* and *Zhimu* both in a large dose clear away heat in *Qi* phase, *Renshen,* *Gancao* and *Jingmi* complement *Qi* and body fluid.

| Application | *Baihu Jia Renshen Tang* has been often used for the treatment of diabetes, type B epidemic encephalitis, epidemic hemorrhagic fever, influenza, viral pneumonia, typhoid, leptospirosis, measles, septicemia, heat stroke and disease with unclear cause, only if intense heat in the *Qi* phase with obvious deficiency of *Qi* and body fluid. |

Article 34

Guizhi Tang syndrome in *Taiyang* pattern has been treated with catharsis erroneously, which causes an incessant diarrhea and hurried pulse, indicating an unrelieved exterior syndrome, and when dyspnea and sweating appear simultaneously, it should be treated mainly by *Gegen Huanglian Huangqin Tang.*

Gegen Qin Lian Tang	*Gegen* 15 g, *Huangqin* 9 g, *Huanglian* 9 g and *Zhi Gancao* 6 g.
Synopsis	The clinical presentations and treatment of diarrhea due to damp-heat in the large intestine complicated with mild exterior syndrome.
Commentary	*Taiyang* wind invasion syndrome should be treated by *Guizhi Tang,* so catharsis therapy brings about an incessant diarrhea that suggests heat with damp pathogen transformed from exterior pathogen invading downward into the large intestine.

Here "hurried pulse" means a rapid and urgent pulse, which indicates the tendency of vital *Qi* to expel pathogen outward and indicates the existence of mild exterior syndrome. Dyspnea and profuse sweating both denote an intense internal heat. The other manifestations in this syndrome may have fever, aversion to wind, thirst, watery, sticky and foul stool, hot sensation in the anus when defecating, abdominal pain with mild tenesmus, scanty-dark urine, red tongue with yellow-greasy coating, and floating-slippery-rapid pulse.

In *Gegen Qin Lian Tang*, *Gegen* expels wind-heat outward to relieve exterior syndrome and lifts clear *Yang* to stop the diarrhea, *Huangqin* and *Huanglian* clear away the heat with damp from the large intestine and lung, and *Zhi Gancao* harmonizes between exterior and interior and eases the urgency. Thus this formula has dual actions, i.e., clearing away heat with damp in both the large intestine and lung, and next, relieving the exterior syndrome, hence being suitable for this syndrome.

Application *Gegen Qin Lian Tang* has been used as a basic formula for acute diarrhea due to heat with damp accumulation in the large intestine regardless of whether exterior syndrome is present, and can be extensively applied in treatment of acute enteritis, chronic colitis, bacterial dysentery, typhoid fever, epidemic encephalitis B, viral encephalitis, measles, pneumonia, aphtha, infantile diarrhea, infantile paralysis syndrome, infection of the upper respiratory tract and so on.

5.3   Deficiency-cold syndromes transmuted from *Taiyang* pattern

——— Article 64 ———

When copious sweating has been induced, the patient's hands are crossed over the precordial region, and there are palpitations with a desire for being pressed, so it should be treated mainly with *Guizhi Gancao Tang*.

Guizhi Gancao Tang	*Guizhi* 12 g and *Zhi Gancao* 6 g.

Synopsis	The principal symptoms and treatment of the palpitations due to heart-*Yang* weakness after excessive induction of sweating.

Commontary	This transmuted syndrome arises from excessive sweating leading to damage of heart-*Yang* since sweat is the body fluid of the heart, so manifested as severe palpitations with a desire for being pressing due to a hollow feeling over the heart location, with the patient's hands crossed over the precordial region. The other symptoms include suffocative chest, shortness of breath, lassitude, pale complexion, spontaneous sweating with cold limbs, and a thready-moderate or knotted-forceless pulse.

Guizhi warms the heart-*Yang* to propel blood flow, acting as sovereign medicine, while *Zhi Gancao* strengthens heart-*Qi* to calm the mind as a minister medicine, both having a special action to warm heart-*Yang* so as to promote blood circulation and relieve palpitations.

Application	*Zhang Zhongjing* used *Guizhi Gancao Tang* as a basic formula for warming heart-*Yang*, and then devised a series of formulas to treat the similar but more serious disorders, such as *Guizhi Gancao Longgu Muli Tang, Ling Gui Zhu Gan Tang, Xiao Jianzhong Tang, Zhi Gancao Tang* and the like. At present, this formula is often used for heart failure in coronary heart disease and rheumatic heart disease, hypotension, cardiac asthma and dysfunction of vegetative nerves.

Article 118

The patient with fidgets caused by fire therapies such as hot-needling and catharsis, should be treated mainly with *Guizhi Gancao Longgu Muli Tang*.

Guzhii Gancao Longug Muli Tang	*Guizhi* 6 g, *Zhi Gancao* 9 g, *Longgu* 15 g and *Muli* 15 g.

| **Synopsis** | The principal symptoms and treatment of weakened heart-*Yang* with a restless heart-mind. |

| **Commentary** | Wrong treatment twice, i.e., hot-needling and catharsis, weakens heart-*Yang* and further aggravates heart-mind restlessness, marked by fidgets, fright-palpitation, timidity, insomnia, profuse sweating, cold limbs, seminal emission, and a thready-weak or knotted pulse. |

In *Guizhi Gancao Longgu Muli Tang, Guizhi* and *Zhi Gancao* warm heart-*Yang* and tonify heart-*Qi, Longgu* and *Muli* astringe *Yang Qi* and calm heart-mind via heavy suppression, so this formula is suitable for such mental disorders caused by deficient heart-*Yang* leading to a restless mind.

| **Application** | *Guizhi Gancao Longgu Muli Tang* has been applied for many disorders due to weak heart-*Yang* with a restless mind in the later ages, including fright-palpitation, timidity, restlessness, insomnia with dreamfulness, hallucinasion, dull expression, spontaneous and night sweating, sperm emission, enuresis, etc., only if their pathogenises present within this syndrome. |

Article 112

Cold-induced disease with floating pulse is treated by fire therapy to enforce sweating, with observed fright, mania, and severe restlessness due to *Yang* floating outward, thus should be treated mainly by *Guizhi Qu Shaoyao Jia Shuqi Muli Longgu Jiuni Tang* (abbreviated as *Guizhi Jiuni Tang*) .

| *Guizhi Jiuni Tang* | *Guizhi* 9 g, *Zhi Gancao* 6 g, *Shengjiang* 9 g, *Dazao* 6 g, *Shuqi* 9 g (decocted first), *Longgu* 12 g and *Muli* 15 g. |

| **Synopsis** | The basic symptoms and treatment of heart-*Yang* floating outward with phlegm leading to severe mental disorders. |

| **Commentary** | Cold-induced disease with floating pulse suggests an exterior syndrome which should be treated by proper diaphoresis; however, it was treated |

wrongly by fire therapy to force sweating, leading to serious damage of heart-*Yang* due to massive sweating, and floating outward of heart-*Yang* leads further to failure to keep the mind housed in the heart; simultaneously, endogenous phlegm also disturbs mind, and is manifested as severe fright, timidity, restlessness, insomnia with nightmares, or even mania, cold sweating with cold limbs, intolerance of cold, shortness of breath, stuffy chest, fatigue, frequent urination, pale tongue with white coating, and a thready-wiry-weak pulse.

In *Guizhi Jiuni Tang*, *Guizhi* and *Zhi Gancao* assisted by *Shengjiang* and *Dazao* warm heart-*Yang* and strengthen heart-*Qi*; *Longgu* and *Muli* calm the mind by heavily suppressing the heart, and stop sweating through astringing action; and *Shuqi* as the sprout of *Changshan*, opens the orifices by removing phlegm to restore the mind. Here, removal of *Baishao* from *Guizhi Tang* is because it has cold in nature and stagnates flow of *Yang-Qi*. Thus this formula is suitable for this syndrome.

Application

Nowadays *Guizhi Jiu Ni Tang* can be used for some severe mental disorders due to deficiency of heart-*Yang* with phlegm clouding the mind, including depressive psychosis and schizophrenia.

In consideration of *Shuqi'* toxicity and difficulty to be obtained, it should be used in a small dose or replaced with the other drugs for removing phlegm to open the orifices and calm the mind, such as *Tiannanxing*, *Shichangpu* and *Tianzhuhuang*.

—— Article 67

After cold-induced disease treated by emesis or catharsis there are an adverse fullness in the epigastric region with upward rushing of *Qi* to the chest, vertigo while getting up, and deep-tense pulse, and should be treated mainly by *Fuling Guizhi Baizhu Gancao Tang*. If it is treated by diaphoresis, the meridian *Qi* will be harassed and the body is shaking.

Ling Gui Zhu Gan Tang	*Fuling* 15 g, *Guizhi* 9 g, *Baizhu* 9 g and *Zhi Gancao* 6 g.

Synopsis

The clinical manifestations and treatment of fluid-retention syndrome in the middle *Jiao* due to weakness of spleen-*Yang* and its contraindication.

Commentary

This syndrome is mainly caused by weakness of spleen-*Yang* leading to fluid-retention in the middle *Jiao*, arising from cold-induced disease treated improperly. Improper emesis or catharsis brings on an impairment of *Yang Qi*, and deficiency of spleen-*Yang*, giving rise to fluid-retention in the middle *Jiao*, then manifesting as fullness-stuffiness in the epigastric region with a vibrating feeling like water waves when palpating the stomach, accompanied by nausea and vomiting. Moreover, the fluid-retention also results in an adverse ascending of *Qi* in the middle *Jiao*, thus there is a special sensation of upward rushing of *Qi* from the abdomen to the chest; if it attacks the heart and lung upward, there will be palpitations, cough with watery sputum, asthma and a suffocative chest; if it clouds the clear orifices in the head, there will be vertigo, deafness and heavy head; and if it flows downward into the intestines, there will be abdominal distention, borborygmus and watery diarrhea. Moreover, pale-puffy tongue with white-slippery coating, and a deep-tense or wiry pulse suggest the fluid-retention within the interior of the body.

Fuling is used as a principal drug for removing fluid-retention by inducing diuresis and invigorating the spleen and heart, *Guizhi* and *Baizhu* warm spleen-*Yang* to transport body fluid and dissipate damp-water, while *Zhi Gancao* strengthens *Qi* and harmonizes all drugs, so the four combined ingredients can warm *Yang* to invigorate the spleen, and expel fluid-retention by promoting urination.

Application

Ling Gui Zhu Gan Tang has been used extensively as a fundamental formula for many diseases in Western medicine, which all belong to the syndrome of fluid-retention resulting from deficiency of spleen-*Yang*, such as chronic gastritis, retention of gastric fluid, dysfunction of autonomous nerves, peptic ulcer, Meniere's disease, chronic bronchitis, bronchial asthma, rheumatic heart disease, pulmonary heart disease, heart failure, chronic nephritis, and so on.

In this formula, *Fuling* should be used in a large amount, usually 15~30 g, and *Gancao* in a small dose, e.g., 3~6 g. Importantly, it can't be used for *Yin* deficiency or intense heat syndrome.

Article 102

Cold-induced disease lasting 2 or 3 days, marked chiefly by palpitations and fidgets, should be treated mainly with *Xiao Jianzhong Tang*.

Xiao Jianzhong Tang	*Yitang* 30 g melting, *Baishao* 18 g, *Guizhi* 9 g, *Shengjiang* 9 g, *Dazao* 6 g and *Zhi Gancao* 6 g.
Synopsis	The main clinical manifestations and treatment of deficiency of both *Yang* and *Yin in the* middle *Jiao*.
Commentary	In the early stage of the exogenously contracted disease, there may be an exterior or excess syndrome, but here palpitations suggesting *Yang* deficiency, and fidgets suggesting *Yin* deficiency, so there must be an interior deficiency syndrome, especially located in the spleen-stomach, without exterior syndrome.

According to the application of *Xiao Jianzhong Tang* by Zhang Zhongjing and the other medical specialists over time, the formula is suitable for the syndrome of deficiency of both *Yang* and *Yin,* but *Yang* deficiency is more serious than *Yin* deficiency, due to hypofunction of the spleen-stomach, and should be treated with nourish *Qi* of the middle *Jiao* first, hence its indications include epigastric or abdominal pain, alleviated by warmth and pressure, poor appetite, cold limbs, dizziness, short breath, lassitude, palpitations, fidgets, insomnia, dry mouth and throat, low fever or feverish sensation in the five centers, pale or sallow complexion, or emaciation, pale-thin tongue with thin coating and a thready-weak or with wiry pulse.

In *Xiao Jianzhong Tang*, *Yitang* (malt sugar) warms and tonifies the spleen-stomach, *Guizhi* and *Shengjiang* warm *Yang* in the middle *Jiao* to unblock meridians, *Baishao* and *Dazao* nourish *Yin*-blood, and are incorporated with *Yitang* and *Zhi Gancao* to relax the tendons and muscles to relieve pain, so the formula possesses the multiple actions of warming *Yang* and nourishing *Yin* by tonifying the spleen-stomach and producing *Qi*-blood, simultaneously relaxing tendons and muscles to relieve spasms and pain.

| Application | *Xiao Jianzhong Tang* and its modifications can be extensively applied to treat a lot of diseases in Western medicine only if they are caused by deficiency of both *Yang* and *Yin* due to hypofunction of the spleen-stomach, such as peptic ulcer, chronic gastritis, prolapse of stomach, chronic hepatitis and cholecystitis, gastrointestinal dysfunction, postpartum abdominal pain, asthenic fever, arrhythmia, neurosis, hemolytic jaundice, etc.. |

Article 66

Abdominal distention and fullness appearing after diaphoresis should be treated mainly with *Houpo Shengjiang Banxia Gancao Renshen Tang.*

| *Houpo Shengjiang Banxia Gancao Renshen Tang* | *Houpo* 12 g, *Shengjiang* 12 g, *Banxia* 12 g, *Zhi Gancao* 6 g and *Renshen* 3 g. |

| Synopsis | The symptoms and treatment of abdominal distention and fullness due to *Qi* stagnation with phlegm-damp retention and *Qi* deficiency in the middle *Jiao*. |

| Commentary | This article mentions only one symptom, abdominal distention-fullness, but its pathogenesis and basic symptoms can be inferred from analysis on the formula applied. In this formula, *Houpo*, *Shengjiang* and *Banxia* in a larger amount can dispel phlegm-damp to propel *Qi* flow in the middle *Jiao*, and *Renshen* and *Zhi Gancao* in a small dose can invigorate the spleen to strengthen *Qi*, so pathogenesis of the syndrome must be *Qi* stagnation in the middle *Jiao* due to phlegm-damp retention with *Qi* deficiency of spleen. This initially arises from improper diaphoresis, and then manifested as abdominal |

distention-fullness intensified in afternoon or after meals, frequent belching and passing gas, poor appetite, nausea or vomiting, listlessness, lassitude, shortness of breath, borborygmus, loose stools but with unsmooth defecation, pale-puffy tongue with white-greasy coating, and a deep-thready-wiry pulse.

Application

Houpo Shengjiang Banxia Gancao Renshen Tang is a formula with actions of dispelling phlegm-damp and supporting spleen-*Qi*, so it can be used for chronic gastrointestinal dysfunction, chronic gastritis and chronic enteritis, marked chiefly by abdominal distention-fullness, and it is caused mainly by *Qi* stagnation due to phlegm-damp retention with *Qi* deficiency.

When applying this formula, *Houpu*, *Shengjiang* and *Banxia* have a larger dose, and *Renshen* and *Gancao* have a smaller dose. Add *Baizhu*, *Fuling* and *Baibiandou* in case of more serious spleen deficiency, and add *Cangzhu*, *Chenpi* and *Sharen* in case of more serious phlegm-damp leading to *Qi* stagnation.

—— Article 61

After catharsis and then diaphoresis, there are fidgets with sleeplessness in the daytime, but quietness at night, no thirst, no vomiting, no exterior syndrome, deep-faint pulse, and no obvious fever, it should be treated mainly by *Ganjiang Fuzi Tang*.

Ganjiang Fuzi Tang

Ganjiang 6 g and raw *Fuzi* 9 g.

Synopsis

The symptoms and treatment of fidgets caused by severe exhaustion of *Yang* after wrongful diaphoresis and catharsis.

Commentary

This is a severe transmuted syndrome resulting from severe *Yang* exhaustion after wrong treatment. Here "fidgets with sleeplessness in the daytime" is because the patient suffering *Yang* exhaustion can get assistance of natural *Yang* in the daytime and then fight against cold pathogen, but "quietness at night" refers to sluggishness due to further depleted *Yang* at night failing to struggle against *Yin*-cold. "No exterior syndrome" indicates an interior syndrome without *Taiyang* pattern, "no thirst" excludes *Yangming* pattern, "no vomiting" excludes *Shaoyang* pattern, a "deep-faint pulse" means a severe deficiency of *Yang*, and "no obvious fever" denotes a false heat symptom arising from excessive *Yin* rejecting *Yang* outward to the body surface.

Raw *Fuzi* and *Ganjiang* together have a very strong action of restoring *Yang* to prevent collapse and save a life, furthermore, concentrated decoction taken once orally can enhance the therapeutic effect of this formula.

Application	*Ganjiang Fuzi Tang* can be seen as *Sini Tang* minus *Gancao* and thus used for some severe disorders with *Yang* about to deplete in the following diseases in Western medicine: edema due to heart failure or nephritis, ascites due to liver cirrhosis, infectious shock, vertigo due to hypotension or hypoglycemia, and Meniere's disease.

———— Article 69 ————

The disease is unresolved after diaphoresis or catharsis, and marked chiefly by restlessness, should then be treated mainly by *Fuling Sini Tang*.

Fuling Sini Tang	*Fuling* 15 g, raw *Fuzi* 9 g, *Ganjiang* 6 g, *Zhi Gancao* 6 g and *Renshen* 3 g.
Synopsis	Principal symptom and treatment of *Yang* exhaustion with *Yin* deficiency due to giving a wrong treatment.
Commentary	Wrongful diaphoresis or catharsis consumes not only *Yang-Qi* but also *Yin*-fluid. The severe restlessness in this syndrome is caused by exhaustion of *Yang* and *Yin* of the heart and kidney due to excessive induction of sweating or purgation, and may be accompanied with aversion to cold, cold limbs, ceaseless cold sweating, shortness of breath, palpitations, dry throat, pale complexion, pale and puffy tounge with white-slippery coating, and a deep-thready or faint pulse.

Fuling Sini Tang can be seen as *Sini Tang* plus *Fuling* and *Renshen*. *Sini Tang* can restore the *Yang* of the heart-kidney to prevent colapse, *Fuling* and *Renshen* tonify *Qi* and *Yin* of the heart to calm the mind, and *Fuling* cooperates with *Fuzi* and *Ganjiang* to remove fluid-retention by promoting urination.

Application	The formula is used for *Yang* exhaustion of the heart and kidney with *Yin* deficiency leading to restlessness, palpitations, suffocative chest, edema, diarrhea, dysuria and frequent urination, which are all seen in Western medicine diseases such as rheumatic heart disease, pulmonary heart disease, cardiac failure, acute and chronic gastroenteritis, colitis and intestinal tuberculosis.

—— Article 82 ——

Taiyang pattern is unrelieved after diaphoresis, and marked by fever, palpitations, vertigo, muscular twitching, and shaking of the body that is about to fall down, and should be treated mainly by *Zhenwu Tang*.

Zhenwu Tang	*Zhi Fuzi* 9 g, *Fuling* 15 g, *Shengjiang* 9 g, *Baizhu* 6 g and *Baishao* 9 g.
Synopsis	The primary symptoms and treatment of *Yang* deficiency of the kidney and spleen with water overflow after excessive diaphoresis.
Commentary	*Taiyang* pattern after undue diaphoresis damaging *Yang Qi* of the heart and kidney has become a transmuted syndrome, marked by an overflowing of water pathogen due to *Yang* deficiency of the kidney and spleen, which leads to retention of body fluid, and then endogenous water pathogen attacking the heart. This brings on palpitations and stuffiness in the chest, clouding the clear *Yang* on vertigo and heaviness in the head, flowing into the muscles and tendons and impeding the distribution of *Yang Qi* along muscles, resulting in twitching and shaking of the body with going to fall down. Here fever arises from deficient *Yang* floating outward. The other manifestations may present dysuria, edema, nausea, vomiting, poor appetite, abdominal distention or dull pain, loose stool, borborygmus, pale-puffy or blackish-lusterless complexion, intolerance of cold, pale-puffy tongue with teeth marks and white-slippery coating, and a deep-thready-weak pulse.

This syndrome can be treated by *Zhenwu Tang,* which has a strong action to warm *Yang* of kidney and spleen in order to remove water retention by promoting urination, because in this formula, *Fuzi* warms kidney-*Yang* to enhance *Qi*-transformation, *Fuling* expels the water pathogen by inducing diuresis, *Baizhu* and *Shengjiang* warm the spleen-*Yang* to dissipate water-damp, and *Baishao* reduces the side effects of *Fuzi*, promotes diuresis and relaxes the tendons to relieve twitching. So this formula can be used for syndrome of *Yang* deficiency leading to overflow of the water pathogen regardless of wrong treatment.

| Application | *Zhenwu Tang* has been presently applied for diseases in Western medicine such as chronic heart failure due to rheumatic heart disease, pulmonary heart disease, hypertension, acute and chronic nephritis, nephrotic syndrome, chronic gastritis, chronic enteritis, prolapse of stomach, chronic bronchitis, bronchial asthma, and pulmonary emphyzema. |

Article 29

Cold-induced disease with floating pulse, spontaneous sweating, frequent urination, fidgets, slight aversion to cold and spasms of lower limbs, treated by *Guizhi Tang* to relieve exterior syndrome, which is a mistake, because it causes cold limbs, dry throat, vexation and vomiting. *Gancao Ganjiang Tang* should be used to restore *Yang*; then we must give *Shaoyao Gancao Tang* to relax the lower limbs after the cold limbs have become warm; if the *Qi* of the stomach-intestine is obstructed, it is occasionally marked by delirium, *Xiao Chengqi Tang* may be given in a small dose; if the second diaphoresis and hot needling are used inappropriately, it should be treated mainly by *Sini Tang*.

| *Gancao Ganjiang Tang* | *Zhi Gancao* 12 g and *Ganjiang* 6 g. |

| *Shaoyao Gancao Tang* | *Baishao* 12 g and *Zhi Gancao* 12 g. |

| Synopsis | Main symptoms and treatment of different transmuted syndromes due to deficiency of both *Yang* and *Yin* in cold-induced disease after wrong |

treatment.

Commentary

The cold-induced disease with spontaneous sweating, slight aversion to cold and floating pulse suggests a *Taiyang w*ind invasion syndrome. However, frequent urination, fidgets and spasms indicate a severe deficiency of both *Yang* and *Yin* in the interior, which cannot be treated wrong by *Guizhi Tang*, because using this formula would lead to more serious deficiency disorders of both *Yang* and *Yin* due to its action of inducing sweating by pungent-warm medicines, such as cold limbs and vomiting resulting from worsening *Yang* deficiency; however, dry throat and vexation from worsening *Yin* deficiency. Generally speaking, *Yang* deficiency is more urgent and invigorating *Yang* can secure *Yin*, so we must use *Gancao Ganjiang Tang* to invigorate *Yang Qi* first, followed by *Shaoyao Gancao Tang* to nourish *Yin*-blood and relax tendons-muscles for relieving spasms and pain. Meanwhile, if wrong treatment gives rise to *Yangming* obstruction syndrome or *Shaoyin* cold-transformation syndrome, *Xiao Chengqi Tang* or *Si Ni Tang* can be used respectively thereby.

Application

Though *Guizhi Tang* belongs to formula with properties of tonifying vital *Qi* and eliminating pathogen, it can be applied for mild deficiency of both *Yang* and *Yin*, but not for an excess syndrome.

Shaoyao Gancao Tang is effective for pain, spasm, rigidity and twitching due to *Yin*-blood deficiency leading to an excessive contraction of the tendons and muscles, thus it is often used in combination with other relevant formulas, and in this case *Baishao* has a large amount dose, of usually more than 30 g.

Article 177

The cold invasion disease marked by a knotted or intermittent pulse, and severe palpitations, should be treated mainly with *Zhi Gancao Tang*.

| *Zhi Gancao Tang* | *Zhi Gancao* 12 g, *Guizhi* 9 g, *Shengjiang* 9 g, *Renshen* 6 g, *Shengdihuang* 50 g, *Maidong* 20 g, *Heizhima* 15 g, *Ejiao* 6 g and *Dazao* 20 g. |

Decoct the 8 herbal medicines with 1200 ml of rice wine and 1300 ml of water to get 360 ml of decoction, then remove the dregs, and melt *Ejiao* into the hot decoction. Afterwards, take 120 ml as the first dose, 3 times a day.

| **Synopsis** | The main manifestations and treatment of deficiency of both heart-*Yin* and heart-*Yang* leading to severe palpitations and arrhythmia. |

| **Commentary** | During the course of exogenous diseases when severe palpitations and a knotted or intermittent pulse appear, it may be caused by several pathogeneses. However, here it must be caused by deficiency in the heart, which fails to be nourished by *Yin*-fluid and *Yang Qi*, but *Yin*-fluid deficiency is more serious according to different doses of all ingredients in *Zhi Gancao Tang*. In addition to above two symptoms, the other symptoms may present stuffy or suffocative chest, fidgets, insomnia, dry mouth and throat, dizziness, pale complexion, shortness of breath, lassitude, and pale or red-delicate tongue with thin-dry coating. |

In this formula, *Zhi Gancao,* as a chief drug, strengthens heart-*Qi* to restore normal rhythm. *Shengdihuang, Maidong, Ejiao, Heizhima* and *Dazao* in larger doses nourish heart-*Yin* to replenish the vessels, and *Guizhi, Shengjiang, Renshen* and rice wine warm heart-*Yang* to boost blood circulation.

| **Application** | *Zhi Gancao Tang* has been extensively applied to a lot of diseases in Western medicine only if there is pathogenesis of deficiency of both *Yin* and Yang of the heart, such as different kinds of arrhythmia (tachycardia, bradycardia, premature beat, ventricular fibrillation or flutter, atrioventricular block, sick sinus syndrome and preexcitation syndrome), viral myocarditis, cardiac insufficiency due to coronary heart disease, rheumatic heart disease and pulmonary heart disease, and cardiac neurosis. While using it to treat these disorders, *Zhi Gancao, Shengdihuang* and *Dazao* are required in large amounts, otherwise, the therapeutic results would be inadequate. |

5.4 Chest-agglomeration syndromes

--- **Article 134** ---

Taiyang pattern is marked with floating-hurried-rapid pulse. Here floating pulse denotes wind, rapid pulse denotes heat, hurried pulse denotes pain, and rapid pulse also denotes shapeless heat pathogen. Meanwhile, there are headache, fever, mild sweating, and aversion to cold, all suggesting that the exterior syndrome has not been relieved yet. When the doctor uses catharsis instead of diaphoresis, the hurried and rapid pulse becomes relatively quiet and slow, and the pain with tenderness around the diaphragm due to the pathogen attacking on the basis of a hollow stomach, manifested as shortness of breath, fidgets, and extreme distress. Furthermore, a heat pathogen that deeply invades into the chest-diaphragm, resulting in hardness in the epigastrium, indicates formation of a chest-agglomeration syndrome, which should be treated mainly with *Da Xianxiong Tang*.

If there is no chest-agglomeration, marked by sweating only on the head above the neck, and no sweating elsewhere, and scanty urine, jaundice may appear.

Da Xianxiong Tang	raw *Dahuang* 18 g, *Mangxiao* 12 g and *Gansui* 1.5 g. Decoct *Dahuang* with 720 ml water first to get 240 ml, then remove the dregs, and put *Mangxiao* into the decoction and boil it for seconds, and afterwards add *Gansui* powder into it. Finally take half of the warm decoction, and stop taking the rest if suddenly diarrhea occurs.

--- **Article 135** ---

After *Taiyang* cold invasion syndrome lasting for 6 or 7days, pathogens agglomerated in the chest-diaphragm, which pertain to an excess and heat syndrome, marked by a deep-tense pulse and epigastric pain with a stony hardness while pressing, and should be treated mainly by *Da Xianxiong Tang*.

Formation, basic pathogenesis, main symptoms and treatment of chest-agglomeration（*Jiexiong* 结胸）syndrome and its difference to *Yang* jaundice, both being transmuted syndromes of *Taiyang* pattern.

Commentary

The Article 134 can be divided into three parts. The first paragraph discusses wind-heat pathogen invading into the exterior body and leading to a wind-heat exterior syndrome, maked by fever, aversion to cold, headache and a floating-rapid pulse. Here mild sweating and a hurried-rapid pulse suggest an intense internal heat but no shaped pathogen within the body.

The second paragraph introduces major chest agglomeration（大结胸）syndrome, in which pathogenic heat and water agglomerate together in the chest and epigastrium due to wrongly catharsis, and belonging to an excess-heat syndrome, manifested as obvious pain and hardness with tenderness in the area around diaphragm, extreme distress or stuffiness with fidgets, shortness of breath or even asthma, fever, profuse sweating, thirst but drinking less, scanty-dark urine, and a deep-tense or slippery-rapid pulse, which is called as major chest-agglomeration syndrome（*Da Xianxiong Zheng* 大陷胸证）and should be treated with *Da Xianxiong Tang*.

In this formula, raw *Dahuang* and *Mangxiao* in a larger dose have a very strong action in removing heat and water pathogens by purgation, and *Gansui* can drastically expel water retention through both urination and defecation.

The third paragraph gives a comparison between *Yang* jaundice and chest-agglomeration, both caused by the heat pathogen deeply invading from the exterior into the interior due to wrong treatment; however, the former refers to heat and damp accumulation in the spleen and liver, leading to obstruction of bile excretion, thus presenting *Yang* jaundice with fever, sweating above the neck, bitter taste in the mouth, nausea, disgust at food, heavy body, scanty-dark urine, red tongue with yellow-greasy coating, and a soft-wiry-rapid pulse.

The Article 135 emphasizes the main pathogenesis, chief symptom and basic formula of the major chest-agglomeration syndrome.

Application *Da Xianxiong Tang* has a very drastical action to eliminate waer retention combined with heat in the chest and abdomen, thus it cannot be used for deficiency-cold syndrome and cannot be used continuously. Presently this formula can be applied for severe cases of acute intestinal obstruction, acute pancreatitis and acute cholecystitis.

Article 137

Taiyang **pattern after repeated diaphoresis and then catharsis, manifested as an inability to defecate for 5 or 6 days, dry tongue, thirst, mild tidal fever at 3~5 o'clock in the afternoon, and hardness-fullness and severe pain expanding from the epigastric region to the lateral-lower abdomen with evident tenderness, should be treated mainly by** *Da Xianxiong Tang.*

Synopsis The primary symptoms and treatment of the severe type of major chest-agglomeration syndrome.

Commentary The severity of major chest-agglomeration syndrome in this article manifests in the following aspects: dry tongue and thirst indicate a more intense interior heat, constipation for 5 or 6 days and tidal fever at 3~5 o'clock in the afternoon suggest intense *Yangming* obstruction syndrome, accompanied with hardness, fullness and serious pain expanding from the epigastric region into the lateral-lower abdomen with evident tenderness, which all show that major chest-agglomeration in this article has been deteriorated in range and degree within the disease. However, the same formula, i.e., *Da Xianxiong Tang*, can be still applied for it because of the same basic pathogenesis.

Article 138

The minor chest-agglomeration syndrome located just below the heart, tenderness when pressing this area, and having a floating-slippery pulse, should be treated mainly with *Xiao Xianxiong Tang*.

Xiao Xianxiong Tang	*Gualou* 20 g, *Banxia* 12 g and *Huanglian* 6 g.
Synopsis	The primary pulse, symptoms and treatment of the minor chest-agglomeration（小结胸）syndrome.
Commentary	The minor chest-agglomeration syndrome is caused by the phlegm and heat agglomerating in the area just below the heart, i.e., the lower chest and epigastrium, so its location is smaller than major chest-agglomeration syndrome. Meanwhile, there is an obvious pain in the affected region when pressing, but no pain or a slight pain when not pressing, indicating that its main symptoms are milder than major one. The other manifestations may be a bitter taste and dryness in the mouth but drinking less, restlessness, nausea or vomiting, upset stomach, or cough and dyspnea with yellow-thick sputum expectorated, unsmooth defecation, red tongue with yellow-greasy coating, and a floating-slippery-rapid pulse.

In *Xiao Xianxiong Tang*, *Gualou* clears away heat and remove phlegm to dissipate agglomeration, *Banxia* dissolves phlegm to lower *Qi*, and *Huanglian* clears heat to normalize the stomach, so this formula has an effective action to remove phlegm-heat from the lower chest and epigastric region to dissipate agglomeration. |
| Application | *Xiao Xianxiong Tang* has been extensively used for many diseases exclusively caused by phlegm and heat agglomerated in the epigastrium or chest, such as acute and chronic gastritis, cholecystitis, bronchitis, pneumonia, pleuritis, coronary heart disease, pulmonary heart disease, hepatitis, pancreatitis, and biliary parasitosis. |

5.5　Epigastric stuffiness syndromes

—— Article 151 ——

Taiyang pattern with floating-tense pulse, treated wrongly by purgation, thus the exterior pathogen invades into the interior, then is tranformed into the epigastric stuffiness syndrome, marked by softness in the affected area while pressing, attributed only to _Qi_ stagnation.

Synopsis	Formation and clinical features of the epigastric stuffiness（ _Wanpi_ 脘痞） Syndrome.

Commentary　　*Taiyang* pattern with a floating-tense pulse suggests a *Taiyang* cold invasion syndrome presents, and should be treated by *Mahuang Tang*. However, if it is treated wrongly by purgation, thus the epigastric stuffiness syndrome forms, resulting from the exterior pathogen invading into epigastric region by seizing the opportunity where *Qi* is deficient in the spleen-stomach, which further leads to *Qi* stagnation in the middle *Jiao*. This syndrome has two clinical features: pathologically, only *Qi* stagnation in the epigastric region without any shaped pathogen associated, thus a feeling stuffy in the area without distention, pain, tenderness or tumor, and absence of hardness in this area.

Application　　This article points out that the epigastric stuffiness syndrome is basically characterized by both *Qi* stagnation in terms of the pathogenesis and a soft sensation only in symptomatology, which have both guided the clinical practice of epigastric stuffiness in the later ages, and made difference from the chest-agglomeration disease.

Article 154

A patient suffering from epigastric stuffiness syndrome, marked by feeling of softness when pressing on the epigastrium and a floating pulse on _Guan_ position, should be treated mainly with _Dahuang Huanglian Xiexin Tang_.

Dahuang Huanglian Xiexin Tang	_Dahuang_ 6 g, _Huanglian_ 3 g and _Huangqin_ 3 g.

These 3 ingredients are soaked in 250 ml of boiled water for several minutes, and the dregs removed, then divide the solution into 2 parts. Take a part orally each time, twice a day.

Synopsis

The primary pulse, symptoms and treatment of heat type of epigastric stuffiness syndrome.

Commentary

The epigastric stuffiness in TCM can be seen as a symptom and a disease, arising from _Qi_ stagnation in the stomach, which results from pathogen attack or _Qi_ deficiency. This article introduces an epigastric stuffiness due to heat pathogen obstructing stomach-_Qi_ and leading to _Qi_ stagnstion, characterized by epigastric stuffiness without pain, and softness when pressing, both suggesting there is no shaped pathogen in the epigastric region; moreover, a floating pulse on the _Guan_ position shows _Yang_ pathogen in the middle _Jiao_. According to the formula used for it, the other symptoms may include vexation, thirst, flushed face, bitter taste and dryness in the mouth, red and sore throat, easy hunger, scanty-dark urine, impeded defecation, red tongue with yellow-dry coating, and a slippery-rapid pulse.

Dahuang Huanlian Xiexin Tang takes _Dahuang_ as a principal drug to guide _Qi_ downward by clearing heat and lowering _Qi_ in _Fu_-organs; Huanglian and _Huangqin_ both in a small dose help _Dahuang_ to clear heat and reduce stuffiness.

Application

In addition to heat type of epigastric stuffiness disease corresponding mainly to gastritis, _Dahuang Huanglian Xiexin Tang_ can now be used for many acute congested diseases, such as hemorrhagic apoplexy, blood-heat pattern of bleeding from nose, mouth, gums, anus and uterus, conjunctivitis, pharyngitis, dermatitis, manic psychosis, epilepsy, hypertension, sores and ulcers in the mouth, acute enteritis and dysentery, and jaundice.

It must be emphasized that the formula used for epigastric stuffiness should be soaked in boiled water for a short time and then taken orally like tea in order to acquire the nature of the herbs instead of their flavor. However, when using the same formula to treat bleeding disorders and other more serious excess-heat syndromes, the ingredients should be decocted with water for a long time.

Article 155

The patient suffering epigastric stuffiness, aversion to cold and sweating, should be treated mainly by *Fuzi Xiexin Tang*.

Fuzi Xiexin Tang

Add *Zhi Fuzi* 6 g into *Dahuang Huanglian Xiexin Tang*. The *Zhi Fuzi* decocted alone with water for a long time, remove the dregs, and put into the decoction of the *Xiexin Tang*, divide it into two parts, then take one part orally, twice a day.

Synopsis

The primary symptoms and treatment of heat type of epigastric stuffiness syndrome with exterior *Yang* deficiency.

Commentary

This is a heat type of epigastric stuffiness accompanied with deficiency of exterior *Yang*, manifested as aversion to cold and spontaneous sweating besides the syndrome in Article 154.

Accordingly *Dahuang Huanglian Xiexin Tang* is still used for clearing stomach-heat to relieve stuffiness, and *Fuzi* is added for warming *Yang* to secure the exterior and dispel cold.

Application

The strong heat natured drugs and strong cold natured drugs are used together in a formula but in different preparations that usually aim at different pathogeneses in complicated syndromes, with other formula examples being *Dahuang Fuzi Tang*, *Xiao Qinglong Plus Shigao Tang*, *Da Qinglong Tang*, *Wumei Wan*, etc., which are effective for complicated syndromes and have been highlightened by TCM researchers and practitioners in recent years.

Fuzi Xiexin Tang can be applied now to treat acute chronic gastritis, chronic colitis, dysentery and hematemesis attributable to interior heat with exterior *Yang* deficiency.

—— **Article 149**

The cold-induced disease lasting for 5 or 6 days with vomiting and fever present, indicates a diagnosis of *Chaihu Tang* syndrome, however a physician gives purgative to treat. If the syndrome still presents, *Chaihu Tang* can be still given. Although the catharsis has already been used, *Chaihu Tang* is an acceptable treatment, and the disorder will be relieved effectively by means of steaming fever with shivering and sweating.

If there is fullness, hardness and pain in the epigastric region, it is called chest-agglomeration, and should be treated mainly by *Da Xianxiong Tang*.

If there is fullness without pain in the epigastric region, it is called epigastric stuffiness syndrome, and cannot be treated by *Chaihu Tang*, and *Banxia Xiexin Tang* is suitable.

Banxia Xiexin Tang	*Banxia* 12 g, *Ganjiang* 9 g, *Huanglian* 3 g, *Huangqin* 9 g, *Renshen* 9 g, *Zhigancao* 9 g and *Dazao* 6 g.
Synopsis	Differentiation among the syndromes of *Shaoyang*, major chest-agglomeration and epigastric stuffiness as well as one treatment of the last syndrome.
Commentary	This article introduces three outcomes of *Shaoyang* pattern treated wrongly by catharsis. *Taiyang* cold invasion syndrome lasting for 5 or 6 days may be usually transformed into the other patterns, in which "vomiting and fever" suggest it is a *Shaoyang* pattern, so *Chaihu Tang* is

suitable for the existence of *Shaoyang* syndrome after giving purgative, and "steaming fever with shivering and sweating" suggests an available reaction where the patient's vital *Qi* expels the pathogen outward after taking *Chaihu Tang*.

Next, when the heat pathogen deeply invades into the interior and agglomerates with the water pathogen in the chest and epigastrium, it is marked chiefly by fullness, hardness and pain with tenderness in this area, and known as major chest-agglomeration syndrome. This can then be treated by *Da Xianxiong Tang*.

When heat pathogen and cold pathogen attacking the stomach respectively downward and upward, thus leading to *Qi* stagnation in the epigastrium mixed with deficiency of stomach-*Qi*, there is a type of epigastric stuffiness syndrome that arises. It is manifested as epigastric stuffiness, vomiting, dry mouth with a little desire for drinking, restlessness, diarrhea with borborygmus, abdominal dull pain, poor appetite, lassitude, pale tongue with yellow or white greasy coating, and a deep and wiry pulse.

This type of epigastric stuffiness syndrome can be cured mainly by *Banxia Xiexin Tang*, in which *Banxia* and *Ganjiang* dispel cold-damp in the intestines; *Huanglian* and *Huangqin* clear away heat in the stomach, both combined to relieve stuffiness in the epigastric region, and *Renshen*, *Dazao* and *Zhi Gancao* strengthen the *Qi* to normalize the stomach, hence this formula is effective for this syndrome.

Application   *Banxia Xiexin Tang* has been used as a basic formula since then for the epigastric stuffiness syndrome due to lower cold with upper heat and deficiency of stomach *Qi,* resulting in *Qi* stagnation in epigastric region.

According to modern clinical research, this formula can be applied for a lot of diseases in western medicine, such as acute and chronic gastritis, enteritis, colitis, peptic ulcer, dyspepsia, gastrointestinal dysfunction, chronic hepatitis, chronic dysentery, and so on, only if cold and heat mixed, or damp-heat accumulates in the middle *Jiao* and stomach *Qi* deficiency.

Article 157

The cold-induced disease relieved after sweating results in a dysfunctional stomach, manifested as epigastric stuffiness and hardness, belching with foul odor of undigested food, water retention in the upper lateral abdomen, thunderous borborygmus in abdomen, and diarrhea, should be treated mainly with *Shengjiang Xiexin Tang*.

Shengjiang Xiexin Tang

Shengjiang 12 g, *Ganjiang* 3 g, *Banxia* 9 g, *Huanglian* 3 g, *Huangqin* 9 g, *Renshen* 9 g, *Zhi Gancao* 9 g and *Dazao* 12 pieces.

Synopsis

The primary symptoms and treatment of the stuffiness syndrome caused by cold-heat obstruction in the epigastric region with deficiency of stomach-*Qi*, water pathogen and food retention .

Commentary

Taiyang exterior syndrome should be relieved after sweating, but there is still disturbance in the stomach, which may be caused by the exterior pathogen deeply invading into the epigastrium and damaging stomach-*Qi* due to inappropriate diaphoresis, and leading to further stagnation and adverse ascending of gastrointestinal *Qi* due to water pathogen and food retention, thus manifested as epigastric stuffiness and hardness, belching with odor of undigested food, loud borborygmus and distention in the lateral abdomen, oliguria, and mild edema of the lower legs, in addition to the symptoms as seen in the *Banxia Xiexin Tang* syndrome in the last article.

Therefore, it can be treated by *Shengjiang Xiexin Tang*, that is *Banxia Xiexin Tang* plus *Shengjiang* 12 g and decreasing the dose of *Ganjiang* from 9 g to 3 g in order to enhance the actions of both dispelling the water retention and removing food retention by warming and invigorating spleen-stomach.

Application

This syndrome is basically the same, but slightly differs from *Banxia Xiexin Tang* syndrome, with water retention and food retention in the gastrointestinal tract, so marked by epigastric stuffiness with hardness, frequent belching out an odor of undigested food or vomiting a sour or bitter fluid, loss of appetite, splashing sounds in stomach, borborygmus in intestines, and watery stools.

Article 158

The *Taiyang* wind invasion syndrome treated wrongly by catharsis, with recurrent bouts of diarrhea per day with undigested food in the feces, thunderous borborygmus in the abdomen, stuffiness, hardness and fullness in the epigastrium, retching and fidgets. However, the physician believes that epigastric stuffiness due to the pathogens remained, and thus gives cathartic once again, then stuffiness gets worse, because this is not combination of heat and feces, the stuffiness-hardness is only due to stomach *Qi* deficiency with adverse ascent of the pathogen, so *Gancao Xiexin Tang* can be used mainly.

Gancao Xiexin Tang	*Zhigancao* 12 g, *Renshen* 9 g, *Dazao* 12 Pieces, *Ganjiang* 9 g, *Banxia* 9 g, *Huanglian* 3 g and *Huangqin* 9 g.
Synopsis	The primary symptoms, pathogenesis and treatment of the epigastric stuffiness syndrome with grave diarrhea due to severe *Qi* deficiency of spleen-stomach.
Commentary	The syndrome in this article is similar to *Banxia Xiexin Tang* syndrome, but it has more serious *Qi* deficiency of spleen-stomach because of prolonged severe diarrhea after giving wrongly catharsis twice, and marked by serious epigastric stuffiness, hardness and fullness, numerous bouts of diarrhea per day with undigested food in the stool, thunderous sounds in the abdomen, retching and fidgets, all which indicate a severer deficiency of *Qi* and *Yin* mixed with *Qi* stagnation and a reversal ascent-descent of spleen-stomach due to pathogenic cold and heat accumunation in the epigastric region. For this reason, a large amount of *Zhigancao* combined with *Renshen* and *Dazao* strengthen *Qi* of spleen-stomach, *Ganjiang* and *Banxia* dispel cold and lower stomach *Qi*, while *Huanglian* and *Huangqin* clear away heat to relieve stuffiness.
Application	*Gancao Xiexin Tang* can be extensively applied for chronic gastroenteritis, colitis, peptic ulcer, dyspepsia, chronic pancreatitis, chronic hepatitis, ulcerative stomatitis, and oculo-oro-genital syndrome (Behcer's disease), assuming they arise from *Qi* deficiency of spleen-stomach with cold and heat accumulation in the epigastric region.

5.6 Doubtful-similar syndromes of a transmuted one

Article 161

The cold invasion syndrome relieved partly after diaphoresis or emesis or catharsis, is still marked by epigastric stuffiness and hardness, and incessant belching, should be treated mainly with *Xuanfu Daizhe Tang*.

Xuanfu Daizhe Tang	*Xuanfuhua* 9 g, *Zheshi* 6 g, *Shengjiang* 15 g, *Zhi Banxia* 15 g, *Renshen* 6 g and *Dazao* 12 pieces.
Synopsis	The primary symptoms and treatment of inceassant belching with epigastric stuffiness caused by phlegm stagnation and *Qi* deficiency in the middle *Jiao*.
Commentary	This syndrome is seen as a doubtful-similar one of *Shengjiang Xiexin Tang* syndrome because of two same main symptoms, ie., epigastric stuffiness-hardness and inceasant belching; however, the former resulting from adverse ascending of *Qi* of the liver and stomach due to phlegm stagnation and stomach *Qi* deficiency, and accompanied by poor appetite, reduced food intake, nausea or vomiting, short breath, coughing up copious sputum and so on; the latter from cold & heat accumulation in the epigastric region leading to *Qi* stagnation with stomach-*Qi* deficiency, fluid and food retention, thus accompanied by belching with odor of undigested food, distention-fullness in the abdomen, thunderous borborygmus, diarrhea, fidgets and bitter taste and dryness in the mouth.

Xuanfu Daizhe Tang can be used for this syndrome because *Xuanfuhua* and *Zheshi* dissolve phlegm and lower *Qi* of the liver and stomach, *Shengjiang* and *Banxia* disperse the phlegm retention downward to normalize stomach, *Renshen*, *Gancao* and *Dazao* together invigorate spleen-stomach to strengthen *Qi*.

Xuanfu Daizhe Tang has been extensively applied for diseases in Western medicine due to phlegm or fluid retention with stomach deficiency, such as gastritis, peptic ulcer, gastric retention, regurgitation of gastric juice, neurogenic vomiting and bronchitis.

—— Article 173 ——

The cold-induced disease, marked by heat in the chest and cold in the abdomen, manifested as abdominal pain and severe nausea, should be treated mainly with *Huanglian Tang*.

Huanglian Tang

Huanglian 9 g, *Ganjiang* 9 g, *Guizhi* 9 g, *Banxia* 9 g, *Renshen* 6 g, *Zhi Gancao* 9 g and *Dazao* 12 pieces.

Synopsis

The primary symptoms and treatment of upper heat and lower cold syndrome with abdominal pain and vomiting.

Commentary

This syndrome can be seen as a doubtful one of the *Banxia Xiexin Tang* syndrome actually due to heat in the chest-stomach and cold in the abdomen-intestine with stomach-*Qi* deficiency, so it presents nausea, vomiting, fidgets, hot sensation in the diaphragm, abdominal pain alleviated by warmth and pressure, cold limbs, diarrhea, lassitude and shortness of breath.

Huanglian Tang is the modified *Banxia Xiexin Tang*, that involves removing *Huangqin*, adding *Guizhi*, increasing the dose of *Huanglian* and decreasing the dose of *Renshen*. Therefore, it is stronger to warm the meridian and dispel the cold to relieve pain, but weaker in action to activate *Qi* flow to reduce stuffiness.

Application

Huanglian Tang has been applied for the treatment of acute and chronic gastritis, gastroenteritis and pancreatitis, peptic ulcer, chronic biliary infection and dysentery.

Syndrome	*Banxia Xiexin Tang* Syndrome	*Huanglian Tang* Syndrome
Pathogenesis	cold and heat stagnation in epigastrium with *Qi* deficiency	Cold in intestines and heat in stomach with *Qi* deficiency
Chief symptoms	Epigastric stuffiness with softness when pressing	Abdominal pain and vomiting
Feature of pathogenesis	Equally serious cold and heat, with *Qi* obstruction	Cold is worse than heat with adverse flow of *Qi*

Article 159

A patient suffering from cold invasion syndrome has an incessant diarrhea and hardness-stuffiness in the epigastric region after taking purgative decoction. Thereafter, he has constant diarrhea after taking *Xie Xin Tang* and then taking purgatives, but the diarrhea worsens after *Li Zhong Wan* is given. Since this formula rectifies the middle *Jiao* only, and the disorder located in the lower *Jiao*, should be treated mainly with *Chishizhi Yuyuliang Tang*. Finally, promoting urination should be used if the diarrhea still persists.

Chishizhi Yuyuliang Tang	*Chishizhi* 30 g and *Yuyuliang* 30 g, both broken and then decocted with water.
Synopsis	Four therapeutic rules for stubborn diarrhea in different transmuted syndromes of *Taiyang* pattern due to wrong treatment.
Commentary	This section discusses the different treatments of stubborn diarrhea in four transmuted syndromes of *Taiyang* pattern due to wrong treatment. First, it can be treated by *Gancao Xie Xin Tang* and like, because this syndrome is marked mainly with epigastric hardness-stuffiness and incessant diarrhea resulting from *Qi* deficiency with cold and heat obstruction in the middle *Jiao*.
	However, it is not relieved after taking the formula due to using the

second purgation. Why does it get worse after taking *Li Zhong Tang?* Because the diarrhea is caused by a disorder located in the lower *Jiao* instead of the middle *Jiao*, so it can be treated mainly with *Chishizhi Yuyuliang Tang*, since the formula can stop diarrhea by warming the large intestine and astringing *Qi* of the lower *Jiao*.

If this formula is still ineffective, it should be treated with diuresis to stop the persistent diarrhea, and can be relieved by means of promoting urination to reduce damp-water in the large intestine.

In *Chishizhi Yuyuliang Tang*, *Chishizhi* warms the large intestine and astringes *Qi*, while *Yuyuliang* astringes *Qi* of the intestine to preserve body fluid, so both in large amounts can be decocted together and are effective for prolonged diarrhea in the deficiency syndrome.

Application	This section shows that the same chief symptom (ceaseless diarrhea) is treated by different therapeutic rules and basic formulas due to different pathogeneses (cold, heat, deficiency, excess or different pathological positions), and reflects that TCM treatment is based on syndrome differentiation, i.e., *Bianzheng Lunzhi*.

Article 156

The epigastric stuffiness after *Taiyang* pattern treated by purgation, is not relieved by *Xie Xin Tang* and the like. If the symptom accompanied with thirst, dry mouth, fidgets and dysuria, should be treated mainly with *Wu Ling San*.

Synopsis	The basic symptoms and treatment of epigastric stuffiness due mainly to internal retention of the water pathogen.
Commentary	A patient with a chief symptom epigastric stuffiness appearing after *Taiyang* pattern treated by wrongful purgation is often seen as its transmuted syndromes, like syndromes of *Dahuang Huanglian Xie Xin Tang, Fuzi Xie Xin Tang, Banxia Xie Xin Tang, Shengjiang Xie Xin Tang*

and *Gancao Xie Xin Tang*, all considered as real stuffiness syndromes caused chiefly by *Qi* stagnation in the middle *Jiao*. However, the symptom of epigastric stuffiness in this article due chiefly to water retention is only considered as a doubtful-similar syndrome instead of commonly acknowledged stuffiness syndrome. The other symptoms in this syndrome include dysuria, dry mouth, thirst and fidgets resulting from water retention in the bladder failing to both distribute upward body fluid and moisten the mouth and heart. *Wu Ling San* can remove damp-water by diuresis and stop diarrhea due to drying of the large intestine.

——— Article 28

After taking *Guizhi Tang* or using purgation, there are still stiff pain in the head and nape, superficial presence of fever, no sweating, epigastric fullness with slight pain, and dysuria, which is treated mainly by *Guizhi* Qu *Gui* Jia *Fuling Baizhu Tang*.

Guizhi Qu Gui jia Fuling Baizhu Tang	*Shaoyao* 9 g, *Zhi Gancao* 6 g, *Shengjiang* 9 g, *Baizhu* 9 g, *Fuling* 9 g and *Dazao* 12 g.
Synopsis	Main symptoms and treatment of *Taiyang* transmuted syndrome due to water retention and stagnation of the meridian-*Qi*.
Commentary	"Dysuria" is a key symptom of the syndrome caused by mistreatment damaging the functions of spleen-*Yang* in transportation of body fluid and then leading to water retention in the interior. The water pathogen obstructs the outward distribution of *Yang Qi* gives rise to superficial presence of fever and no sweating; it intrudes into the middle *Jiao* and resulting in *Qi* stagnation of the stomach, so manifested as epigastric fullness with slight pain; and it also impedes *Taiyang* meridian-Qi, thus presenting stiff pain in head and nape.

Why is the syndrome treated by modified *Guizhi Tang*? Because the syndrome is caused by deficiency of both *Yang Qi* and *Yin* blood due to wrong treatment. Adding *Baizhu* and *Fuling* helps *Shengjiang* to warm spleen-*Yang*, dispel water retention and restore flow of *Yang Qi*; meanwhile, *Baishao, Dazao* and *Zhi Gancao* nourish *Yin* blood and relax tendons to relieve pain. However, removing *Guizhi* is for both lack of exterior syndrome and deficiency of *Yin* fluid after mistreatment.

| Application | This formula has the actions of warming *Yang* to invigorate the spleen and expelling water by diuresis, and can be used for influenza and epilepsy due to spleen deficiency and water retention with obstruction of *Yang Qi*, marked by headache, vertigo, stuffy nose, low fever with or without aversion to cold, distending or full stomach, dysuria, nausea and so on. *Guizhi* may be kept in case of a more obvious exterior syndrome; add *Zhuling* and *Zexie* in case of more serious water retention; add *Banxia* and *Chenpi* in case of severer nausea and vomiting; and add *Houpu* and *Xingren* in case of cough and dyspnea. |

—— **Article 152** ——

Taiyang **wind invasion syndrome with diarrhea and vomiting can be purged if the exterior syndrome has been relieved. When the patient has paroxysmal profuse sweating, headache, stuffiness, hardness and fullness in the chest-diaphragm, pulling pain in hypochondriac region, retching, dyspnea, and sweating without aversion to cold, all mean an interior disharmony and although the exterior syndrome has been relieved, it should be treated mainly with *Shi Zao Tang*.**

| *Shi Zao Tang* | *Dazao* 10 pieces, *Yuanhua* 0.5 g, *Gansui* 0.5 g, *Daji* 0.5 g. First decoct *Dazao* with 300 ml of water to get 160 ml, remove the dregs, then put the mixed powder of the other 3 drugs into the decoction, and take it warmly in the morning. If diarrhea is less and the symptoms unrelieved, add 0.5 g powder and take it with the decoction again the next day. The patient should eat rice porridge for recovery as soon as a smooth diarrhea occurs. |

| Synopsis | The manifestations and treatment of severe water-retention in the pleural-hypochondriac region and its difference from the major chest-agglomeration syndrome. |

The first paragraph of this article highlights a general therapeutic sequence while both exterior syndrome and interior fluid-retention syndrome happen simultaneously.

The Main idea of this section lies in the second paragraph. A shaped pathogen, fluid-retention, combined with heat pathogen in the pleural-hypochondriac region (or area arround diaphragm). The fluid-retention and heat pathogen together stagnate *Qi* flow in this area and lead to an adverse ascending of lung-*Qi*, and is therefore manifested as epigastric stuffiness, hardness and fullness, hypochondriac pulling pain, cough and dyspnea with inability to lie flat and expectoration of sputum. The pathogens stay in the stomach, bringing about retching or vomiting, and they obstruct the clear orifices upward, so headache and vertigo appear. If interior heat enforces body fluid discharging outward, so presents much sweating, and no aversion to cold indicates the exterior syndrome has been relieved.

Application

Shi Zao Tang is a famous formula for drastically expelling water and fluid-retention in the interior, especially in the lung and pleural cavity, and can therefore be applied to the following diseases in Western medicine such as exudative pleurisy, ascites and edema belonging to severe excess-heat syndrome. It should be used cautiously and temporarily because of its drastic and toxic action.

Article 166

The disorder resembling *Guizhi Tang* syndrome, without headache and stiff nape, slightly floating pulse on *Cun* position, stuffiness-hardness in the thorax, feeling of *Qi* rushing upward to the throat and dyspnea, all suggest fluid-retention in the chest, and emesis should be induced with *Guadi San*.

Guadi San

Guadi (baked and changed into yellow color) and *Chixiaodou* in equal doses, pound both into fine powder by means of sifting, and then mix them. The powder 3 g and *Dandouchi* 10 g are decocted with 150 ml water into porridge, and then take it warmly once after remove the dregs. Add a little more dose and take it again in case of no vomiting until the patient vomits smoothly. The formula is contraindicated for deficiency syndromes and heavy bleeding cases.

Synopsis

The pathogenesis, main manifestations and treatment of fluid-retention in the thorax (including esophagus) with an ascending trend.

Commentary

"the disorder resembling *Guizhi Tang* syndrome" indicates the disorder with fever, aversion to cold and sweating, so similar to *Taiyang* wind invasion syndrome, but no headache, no stiff nape and floating pulse on *Cun* portion instead of whole *Cunkou*, suggesting it differs from that syndrome. Its main symptoms are stuffiness-hardness in the thorax, feeling of *Qi* rushing upward to the throat, and dyspnea, all showing stagnation of fluid-retention in the thorax with an ascending trend, so emesis is used for expelling the pathogen upward so as to follow the pathological trend, thus *Guadi San* is suitable.

Guadi and *Chixiaodou* together induce vomiting due to their extreme sour and bitter flavors, and *Dandouchi* assists their emesis due to its action of dispersing pathogen upward. Therefore, this formula is thought of as a strong emetic in TCM.

Application

As a typical and representative emetic, *Guadi San* is applied only for excess syndrome caused by shaped pathogen stagnated in the throat, esophagus and stomach, cannot be used for any deficiency syndrome and pathogen stagnated in the lower Jiao. Besides, *Guadi* is toxic. Thus the formula can be only used once or twice.

Article 58

Any disease after diaphoresis, emesis, purgation, hemorrhage, or losing body fluid, can be relieved spontaneously by means of self-regulation of *Yin* and *Yang* within the human body.

Article 59

Dysuria after drastic purgation followed by diaphoresis is due to loss of body fluid. Do not treat it hastily as it may be relieved spontaneously after achieving a smooth urination.

Article 93

Taiyang syndrome is not relieved after purgation, and after inducing sweating again, so resulting in vertigo or even fainting due to deficiency of both the exterior and interior. The patient may recover after spontaneously sweating which denotes a harmonized exterior body. It should be further purged if the interior is still in disharmony.

Article 94

Taiyang syndrome unrelieved and marked by a hidden pulse on three portions of *Cun*, *Guan* and *Chi*, can be relieved after cold shivering followed by sweating. It can be relieved following sweating in case of a weak pulse felt only on *Cun* portion; and it can be relieved after purgation in case of a weak pulse felt only on *Chi* portion, then *Tiaowei Chengqi Tang* is suitable for it.

A lot of diseases and *Taiyang* syndromes can be relieved spontaneously by self-regulation of *Yin* and *Yang* within the body or relieved by using an appropriate remedy.

Commentary

"Self-regulation of *Yin* and *Yang*" is a very important academic thought in TCM, which signifies an ability existing in the human body to adapt itself to environmental changes and adjust the vital activities for resisting various pathogens or reducing the harmful reactions of the pathogens by regulating *Yin* and *Yang* in the body. This is why some diseases can be relieved spontaneously without any treatment. With respect to concrete manifestations of this internal mechanism, there are sweating, urination, vertigo, syncope and shivery sweating (*Zhanhan* 战汗, namely, cold shivering before much sweating) according to these four articles, others include vomiting, fever, aversion to cold, sneezing, cough, diarrhea and so forth.

Furthermore, the ability of self-regulating *Yin* and *Yang* within the human body is not limitless, so TCM treatment is its necessary supplement in severe cases, for example, diaphoresis, purgation and *Tiaowei Chengqi Tang* are used for the exterior and interior disfunction even after other treatment in Article 93 and 94.

Application

Regulating *Yin* and *Yang* can be seen as the highest principle in health-preserving and TCM treatment. However, the therapeutic regulation of *Yin* and *Yang* by a doctor is passive, while self-regulation of *Yin* and *Yang* within the body is active. Therefore, the latter is more valuable than the former, and the TCM doctor should grasp and protect patient's ability of self-regulation of *Yin* and *Yang* and then devise an appropriate treatment scheme.

Questions for Review and Thinking

1. What are basic pathogenesis, main symptoms, therapeutic rules and major formula in *Taiyang* wind invasion syndrome?

2. What disorders can be treated by *Guizhi Tang*? Why?

3. What main concomitant syndromes does *Taiyang* wind invasion syndrome present? How to treat them respectively?

4. What are the main differences between *Taiyang* wind invasion syndrome and *Taiyang* cold invasion syndrome in terms of pathogenesis, manifestations, therapeutic rule and major formula?

5. Try to make a comparison between *Xiao Qinglong Tang* and *Da Qinglong Tang* in pathogenesis, chief symptoms and therapeutic principle.

6. How to distinguish *Taiyang* water retention syndrome and *Taiyang* blood retention syndrome in pathogenesis, main symptoms, therapeutic rule and basic formula?

7. *Ma Xing Gan Shi Tang* and *Gegen Qin Lian Tang* are used for simultaneous exterior and interior syndromes, what are their different pathogegesis, chief symptoms and therapeutic principles?

8. *Gui Gan Long Mu Tang*, *Ganjiang Fuzi Tang*, *Ling Gui Zhu Gan Tang* and *Zhenwu Tang* are all applied for *Yang* deficiency syndromes, how to distinguish them in pathogenesis and key symptoms?

9. *Xiao Jianzhong Tang* and *Zhi Gancao Tang* can tonify both *Yin* and *Yang*. What are different pathogenesis and indications between them?

10. What are main differences between a major chest-agglomeration syndrome and a minor one?

11. What does epigastric stuffiness syndrome mean in *Shanghan Lun*? How to differentiate *Banxia Xie Xin Tang*, *Shengjiang Xie Xin Tang* and *Gancao Xie Xin Tang* in pathogenesis and symptoms?

12. Try to make a comparison between *Banxia Xie Xin Tang* and *Xuanfu Daizhe Tang* in their chief symptoms and pathogenesis.

Chapter II

Differentiation of Symptoms, Pulses and Treatment of *Yangming* Pattern

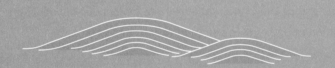

Outlines of *Yangming* Pattern

Article 180

Yangming pattern is marked essentially by the gastrointestinal excess-heat.

| Synopsis | A brief generalization of the basic pathogenesis of *Yangming* pattern. |

Commentary

This article is seen as an outline of *Yangming* pattern caused by an intense dryness-heat pathogen in the interior body, especially in the gastrointestinal tract. The pattern is mainly divided into two principal syndromes, *Yangming* heat syndrome（*Yangming Rezheng* 阳明热证）and *Yangming* obstruction syndrome（*Yangming Shizheng* 阳明实证）. The former refers to dryness-heat pathogen intensifying in both the interior and exterior body, thus marked by high fever, heavy sweating, severe thirst and a surging-rapid pulse; the latter refers to interior heat combined with dry stools obstructing *Qi* of the large intestine, so marked by some specific pathological features, such as stuffiness, fullness, dryness, heat and solidness.

Application

This article deeply reflects the pathlogical essence of *Yangming* pattern in cold-induced disease, i.e., excess and heat in the interior, especially in the stomach and large intestine, which is considered to be the biggest difference between *Yangming* pattern and the other five patterns pathologically.

Article 182

What are the external manifestations of *Yangming* pattern? They includee generalized fever, sweating, and aversion to heat instead of cold.

Synopsis

The primary external symptoms of *Yangming* pattern.

Commentary	Here, "external manifestations of *Yangming* pattern" mean outward appearances resulting from intense excess heat in the interior, especially in the gastrointestinal tract, such as higher fever, aversion to heat, much sweating, flushed face and so on, which are different from the exterior syndrome of *Taiyang* pattern. Of course, they also differ from the internal manifestations of *Yangming* pattern mentioned later.

Application	This article is helpful for syndrome differentiation in the exogenous disease, and is seen as one of the main differences between the exterior syndrome and interior excess heat syndrome.

Article 185

At the beginning of *Taiyang* pattern if diaphoresis is incomplete it may be transformed into *Yangming* pattern. Initially, the cold invasion syndrome should have fever without sweating, and vomiting with inability to eat, but now there is continuously profuse sweating suggesting that there has been a transformation into *Yangming* pattern.

Article 183

Why are there no fever and aversion to cold after one day of suffering a cold-induced disorder? Although one suffers the disease for only one day, there may be spontaneous sweating and aversion to heat after the disappearance of the aversion to cold.

Article 186

Three days after the cold-induced disorder, a surging pulse appears in the *Yangming* pattern.

Synopsis

A possible cause, main pulse and symptoms of *Yangming* heat syndrome transformed from *Taiyang* pattern.

Commentary

Yangming pattern may have multiple causes, such as self-development of an exogenous disease, transformation of *Taiyang* or *Shaoyang* pattern due to delayed or wrong treatment, due to an incomplete diaphoresis to treat the *Taiyang* pattern, here manifested as high fever with continuous excessive sweating, aversion to heat instead of aversion to cold, thirst and a surging-rapid pulse, all indicating formation of *Yangming* pattern, namely *Yangming* heat syndrome.

Application

"Continuously profuse sweating" with fever and aversion to heat can be used as a keypoint for differentiation between *Yangming* heat syndrome and *Taiyang* pattern. Furthermore, aversion to cold or heat, and a floating or surging pulse are thought of two key points distinguishing between the exterior syndrome and interior heat syndrome.

—— Article 181 ————

How to contract a *Yangming* pattern? When *Taiyang* pattern is mistreated by wrong diaphoresis, or purgation, or diuresis, this leads to consumption of body fluid, and to further dryness-heat in the gastrointestinal tract; then, *Yangming* pattern transformed, marked by constipation, obstruction of intestinal *Qi* and difficult defecation, which are called the *Yangming* pattern.

Synopsis

Possible causes, basic pathogenesis and manifestations of *Yangming* obstruction syndrome transformed by the mistreatment of *Taiyang* pattern.

Commentary

Mistreatment of *Taiyang* pattern is a commonly seen cause for formation of *Yangming* pattern, which leads to dryness-heat in the stomach and large intestine due to severe consumption of body fluid, and further brings about an obstruction of the large intestine caused by internal heat and dry stool aggregation, thus marked chiefly by constipation or difficult defecation, with abdominal fullness or distending pain and tenderness, fever, thirst, restlessness and so forth; this is known as *Yangming* obstruction syndrome.

Application	The article displays a pathological essence of *Yangming* obstruction syndrome, that is, internal heat and dry stool aggregated in the large intestine leading to severe obstruction of intestinal *Qi*, marked chiefly by constipation with abdominal fullness, distention and pain, thus belonging to an excess-heat syndrome and also seen as the *Yangming* heat syndrome plus symptoms due to intestinal obstruction.

—— Article 210 ——

The excess syndrome is featured with delirium, and unconscious murmuring in the deficiency one. Unconcious murmuring means repeated speaking the same words. Delirium and staring suggest impending death in case of accompanying dyspnea with suffocation or ceaseless diarrhea.

—— Article 211 ——

Excessive or repetitive induction of sweating can cause *Yang* exhaustion and delirium, which signify a death syndrome in case of very short pulse, or a better prognosis in case of a gradually harmonized pulse.

Synopsis	Differential diagnosis and prognosis of delirium.
Commentary	Since delirium is a common symptom in *Yangming* pattern, especially in *Yangming* obstruction syndrome, these two articles discuss syndrome differentiation and prognosis of this symptom. Generally speaking, delirium（*Zhanyu* 谵语）refers to loud, continuous and unreasonable speech accompanied with high fever, thirst, restlessness or even coma, polypnea and slippery-rapid pulse, which belongs to excess-heat syndrome, caused by intense interior heat or phlegm-heat disturbing the

mind; However, unconscious murmuring（*Zhengsheng* 郑声）refers to low, intermittent and unconscious speech with the repetitive words, accompanied by listlessness, tiredness, shortness of breath, dizziness and a weak or faint pulse, which belongs to a serious deficiency syndrome, caused by depletion of essence-*Qi*.

Staring（*Zhishi* 直视）caused by severe liver-wind syndrome, dyspnea with suffocation indicates serious obstruction of lung-*Qi*, and ceaseless diarrhea denotes a heavy decline of the spleen, so all indicate a critical condition if occurring with delirium.

Moreover, *Yang* exhaustion also leads to delirium due to mental confusion resulting from exhausted heart-*Yang* floating outward, in such circumstances, it is better if the pulse can be restored normally.

| Application | The discussion on delirium, unconscious murmuring and the other accompanying symptoms altogether can give us some ways to think and differentiate syndrome and also prognose disease. |

Section 2 | *Yangming* Heat Syndromes

Article 176

A cold-induced disease with floating and slippery pulse suggests that a heat pathogen is present in both the exterior and interior body, and should be treated mainly by *Baihu Tang*.

| *Baihu Tang* | *Shigao* 50 g, *Zhimu* 18 g, *Jingmi* 30 g and *Zhi Gaqncao* 6 g |
| Synopsis | The primary pathogenesis, manifestations and treatment of *Yangming* heat syndrome. |

This is a typical *Yangming* heat syndrome due to intense heat in both the interior and exterior body, with slight impairment of *Qi* and body fluid, is manifested as high fever, aversion to heat, much sweating, severe thirst with preference for cold drinks, restlessness, flushed face, red tongue with yellow-dry coating, and a surging or slippery-rapid pulse. Therefore, it should be treated by clearing away heat in the *Qi* phase first with tonifying body fluid and *Qi*, here *Baihu Tang* is a basic formula.

In *Baihu Tang*, *Shigao* and *Zhimu* are both in large amounts and have a strong action to clear away the heat pathogen in the whole body, *Jingmi* and *Gancao* strengthen *Qi* and nourish body fluid, thus constituting the strongest formula with a pungent-cold quality.

Application

Baihu Tang is not only used for *Yangming* heat syndrome in cold-induced disease, but also used for the warm-heat pathogen in the *Qi* phase of warm disease. According to the modern pharmocological research and clinical reports, this formula possesses antipyretic, anti-inflammatory, antiviral, anti-allergic, sedative and hypoglycemic effects, thus is extensively applied for such diseases as diabetes, sunstroke, infant heat stroke syndrome, headache, rheumatic fever and schizophrenia.

Article 219

Concurrent occurrence of the three *Yang* patterns marked by abdominal fullness, heavy body with difficulty to move around, loss of sense of taste, dirty face, sometimes delirium and enuresis, should be treated mainly with *Baihu Tang* in case of spontaneous sweating. The delirium worsens in case of diaphoresis, and sweating on the forehead and cold limbs in case of purgation.

Synopsis

Main symptoms and treatment of concurrent occurrence of the three *Yang* patterns with stress on *Yangming* heat syndrome.

Commentary

Concurrent occurrence of two or three patterns should be treated usually by remedies aiming at the two or three patterns simultaneously, however, main symptoms in this article indicate that *Yangming* heat syndrome is a leading one and other two *Yang* patterns are secondary. Why? Here, abdominal fullness and heavy body with difficulty to move around are due to intense interior heat obstucting *Qi* flow and then stagnation of *Qi*-blood; upward flaming of stomach-heat leads to declined taste sensation in the mouth and massive sweats on the face, manifested as loss of taste sense and dirty face; and interior heat disturbing mind upward with heart-spirit losing control consciousness and urination, so sometimes delirium and enuresis occur. Moreover, great spontaneous sweating suggests that intense heat pathogen in *Yangming* forms the first pathogenesis, the *Taiyang* and *Shaoyang* syndromes are less evident. Therefore, *Baihu Tang* is suitable for this syndrome, and diaphoresis and purgation may deteriorate the disorder, resulting from an intensified pathogen or exhausted vital *Qi*.

Application

The article tells us an important principle for treating the concurrent occurrence of several syndromes, i.e., choosing and treating a leading syndrome first which occupies a decisive position among all the others, and thus can determine the success or failure of the treatment.

Article 168

The cold invasion disease after emesis or catharsis has been not relieved for 7 or 8 days, marked by heat accumulation in the interior, and present heat in both exterior and interior body, sometimes aversion to wind, great thirst, dry tongue, fidgets and a desire for drinking much, should be treated mainly by *Baihu Jia Renshen Tang*.

Baihu Jia Renshen Tang

add *Renshen* 6 g into *Baihu Tang*.

Article 169

There is no progressive fever, but presents severe dry mouth with thirst, restlessness, occasionally slight aversion to cold on the back, and should be treated mainly by *Baihu Jia Renshen Tang*.

Article 170

A cold-induced disorder with floating pulse, fever and no sweating cannot be treated by *Baihu Tang* due to unrelief of the exterior syndrome. If thirst with desire for drinks occurs without exterior syndrome, this should be treated mainly with *Baihu Jia Renshen Tang*.

Synopsis	The primary pathogenesis, symptoms and treatment of *Yangming* heat syndrome with obvious damage of *Qi* and body fluid.
Commentary	The syndrome in these three articles discusses longstanding *Yangming* heat syndrome, mixed with a serious deficiency of *Qi* and body fluid. But how to recognize it? First, fever is not very high and there is no progressive fever suggest *Qi* inadquacy due to excessive sweating; secondly, more pronounced thirst with drinking a large amount of water shows intense interior heat severely damaging the body fluid; thirdly, sometimes aversion to wind or occasionally slight aversion to cold on the back results from deficiency of *Qi*, especially defensive *Qi*, caused by massive sweating.
	For this reason, *Renshen* is added into *Baihu Tang* to both strengthen *Qi* and complement body fluid.
Application	*Baihu Jia Renshen Tang* has been used for the same diseases treated by *Baihu Tang* mentioned in last article, but only due to more serious deficient *Qi* and body fluid.

Article 228

In *Yangming* pattern after catharsis, there is a feverish feeling in the external body with warm limbs, extreme distress and fidgets in the chest, hunger with upset stomach and eating less, but without signs of chest-agglomeration, and sweating seen only on the head, it should be treated mainly by *Zhizi Chi Tang*.

Synopsis	The basic symptoms and treatment of *Yangming* pattern after catharsis

marked by mild heat disturbing in the chest-diaphragm.

Commentary *Yangming* pathogen after catharsis, but presence of the residual heat pathogen disturbing in the chest and diaphragm, marked by extreme distress and fidgets, insomnia, feverish feeling in the chest, bitter taste and dryness in the mouth. Here "no signs of chest-agglomeration" means no hardness and pain when pressing the chest-diaphragm because of only shapeless heat pathogen without shaped phlegm or water pathogen; "hunger with upset stomach and eating less" is due to residual and mild heat pathogen in the stomach; and "sweating only on the head" results from upward rushing of heat pathogen in the upper *Jiao*.

Application seeing the same formula in Article 76, Section 5 of Chapter Ⅰ.

Article 223

When a patient displaying a floating pulse, fever, thirst with a desire to drink water and dysuria, should be treated mainly by *Zhuling Tang*.

Zhuling Tang *Zhuling* 9 g, *Fuling* 9 g, *Zexie* 9 g, *Huashi* 9 g and *Ejiao* 9 g.

First decoct the previous 4 drugs with 500 ml of water to get 200 ml. Next remove the dregs and melt *Ejiao* into the hot decoction, and then take 70 ml of the decoction orally each time, 3 times per day.

Synopsis The basic manifestations and treatment of mild *Yangming* heat syndrome with water retention and *Yin* deficiency in the lower *Jiao*.

Commentary This is a concomitant syndrome of mild *Yangming* heat syndrome with water retention and mild *Yin* deficiency, thus marked by fever, thirst with a desire to drink water, dysuria, and a floating-thready-rapid pulse. The other symptoms are distending pain in the lower abdomen, yellow or bloody urine with unsmooth-painful urination, restlessness, insomnia, or nausea, vomiting, diarrhea, red tongue with yellow-greasy coating.

The syndrome should be treated by inducing urination to dispel water retention first, followed by clearing heat and nourishing *Yin*. In *Zhuling Tang, Zhuling, Zexie, Huashi* and *Fuling* remove water and heat by diuresis, while *Ejiao* nourishes *Yin*, so it is suitable for this complicated syndrome.

Application | *Zhuling Tang* has been used for a lot of diseases in Western medicine, such as acute and chronic pyelonephritis, ureteritis, cystitis and urephritis, nephritis, hematuria with unclear cause, liver cirrhosis in the later stage, renal edema, chynuria and kidney stone, all caused by the same pathogenesis mentioned-above.

Section 3 *Yangming* Obstruction Syndromes

Article 248

After *Taiyang* pattern lasting for 3 days, there is no relief although it has been treated by diaphoresis, and is marked by steaming fever from the interior to the exterior, which indicates formation of *Yangming* obstruction syndrome has formed, so should be treated mainly by *Tiaowei Chengqi Tang.*

Article 249

Taiyang cold invasion syndrome after emesis, marked by abdominal distention and fullness, may be relieved by taking *Tiaowei Chengqi Tang.*

Article 207

Yangming pattern not treated by emesis and purgation, but fidgets, *Tiaowei Chengqi Tang* is suitable.

Tiaowei Chengqi Tang	*Dahuang* 12 g, *Zhi Gancao* 6 g and *Mangxiao* 15 g. Decoct the previous two drugs in 360 ml of water to get 120 ml decoction, and remove the dregs, then add *Mangxiao* into it, and decoct it again with boiling once or twice, finally take the whole warm decoction at once to regulate stomach-*Qi*.
Synopsis	Basic symptoms and treatment of *Yangming* obstruction syndrome with evident interior heat and less *Qi* stagnation.
Commentary	This syndrome may result from three ways, *Taiyang* pattern treated by improper diaphoresis, by improper emesis and by heat pathogen directly invading into *Yangming*. The pathological feature is intense heat with dry stool obstructing the intestine in an early stage, i.e., the heat flaming upward is obvious but obstruction of intestinal *Qi* is relatively mild, so presenting steaming fever, fidgets, thirst, abdominal distention, dry stools or constipation, flushed face with congested eyes, or ulcers and sores in the mouth, painful and swollen throat, red tongue with yellow-dry coating, and a slippery-rapid pulse. *Tiaowei Chengqi Tang* belongs to moderate purgatives, since *Mangxiao* and *Dahuang* together have a strong action to the clear heat pathogen for normalizing stomach and soften hardness by moistening dryness, while *Gancao* strengthens *Qi* and slows down the drastically purgative action of the others.
Application	*Tiaowei Chengqi Tang* has a strong action for antipyrexia, antibiosis and detoxication, therefore often used for acute pancreatitis, gallbladder stone, diabetes, ulcerative stomatitis and so on.

Article 213

In *Yangming* syndrome with massive sweating, there will be dryness in the gastrointestinal tract due to outward loss of body fluid, thus the stools becomes hard, and delirious speech follows. It should be treated mainly with *Xiao Chengqi Tang*. If the delirious speech stops after taking the decoction once, there is no need to continue taking it.

Xiao Chengqi Tang	*Dahuang* 12 g, *Zhishi* 15 g and *Houpo* 6 g.
	Decoct the above 3 drugs with 480 ml of water to get 160 ml, then remove the dregs and take half of the decoction warm twice per day. If there is bowel movement after taking the first dose. There is no need to take it any more; if there is no defecation, then the other half may be taken.

Article 214

Yangming pattern marked by delirium, tidal fever in the afternoon, and a slippery and hurried pulse, should be treated mainly with *Xiao Chengqi Tang*. If there is flatulence with borborygmus after taking the first half of the decoction, the other half can be taken; when such symptom dosen't appear, don't take it again. It would be difficult to treat when constipation with faint and an unsmooth pulse appears again the next day, suggesting an interior deficiency syndrome; *Chengqi Tang* and like can't be used.

Synopsis	The primary symptoms, treatment and contraindication of *Yangming* obstruction syndrome with evident *Qi* stagnation and less dryness-heat.
Commentary	This is a middle degree of *Yangming* obstruction syndrome, characterized with severe *Qi* stagnation but mild dryness-heat in the intestines on the basis of inference from the formula used for it. So its main symptoms are abdominal stuffiness, fullness, and distending pain with tenderness, constipation or unsmooth defecation, frequent passing gas, tidal fever in the afternoon, dark-red tongue with yellow-thick-greasy coating, and a slippery-rapid or a deep-forceful pulse. Here, delirium is caused by

turbid-heat pathogen attacking upward and clouding the heart mind, and tidal fever means fever that is intensified at 3–5 pm（*Ribu Chaore* 日晡潮热）due to heat and dry stool together obstructing intestinal *Qi*.

In *Xiao Chengqi Tang*, *Zhishi* and *Houpo* lower intestinal *Qi* to promote defecation, *Dahuang* clears heat by purgation, and altogether can lower intestinal *Qi* to propel bowel movement, and furthermore, clear heat by purgation.

Application
Xiao Chengqi Tang is considered a mild purgative in TCM, and has a strong antispasmodic, choleretic and cathartic actions, thus extensively used for such diseases as intestinal obstruction, complication after surgery for enteroparslysis, ascariasis of biliary tract and irritable bowel syndrome.

Article 239

A patient presents no bowel movement for 5 or 6 days, pain around the navel and paroxysmal restlessness, all suggest dry stools in the abdomen leading to constipation.

Article 215

Yangming pattern marked by delirious speech, tidal fever but with inability to eat food, implies that there must be 5 or 6 pieces of dry stools in the large intestine, so *Da Chengqi Tang* can be used appropriately for expelling them downward. If the patient is able to eat food, there are only hardened stods.

Article 241

After drastic purgation, there are no bowel movement for 6 or 7 days, with fidgets unrelieved, and abdominal fullness and pain, which indicate dry stool in the intestine, originating from food retention, thus *Da Chengqi Tang* is suitable.

Article 255

Abdominal fullness with no diminution or no evident decrease, should be treated by catharsis and then by using *Da Chengqi Tang* appropriately.

Article 238

Yangming pattern after catharsis, manifested still as an extreme distress with vexation in the heart, and when dry stool in the intestine can be confirmed, this can be treated by purgation, and *Da Chengqi Tang* is used appropriately. When there is slight fullness in the abdomen, and hard stool seen at the beginning and loose stools seen later, purgation shouldn't be used.

Da Chengqi Tang	Dahuang 12 g, *Houpo* 20 g, *Zhishi* 15 g and *Mangxiao* 6 g.
	Decoct *Zhishi* and *Houpo* in 1200 ml of water first to obtain 600 ml of decoction, then remove the dregs, next add *Dahuang* into the decoction, and decoct it again to get 240 ml, remove the dregs, then put *Mangxiao* into the decoction for several miniutes of boiling. Take half of the warm decoction twice a day, and cease taking the rest if there is diarrhea after taking the first dose.
Synopsis	The differentiation and treatment of severe *Yangming* obstruction syndrome due to both intense dryness-heat and heavy *Qi* stagnation in the gastrointestinal tract.

These five articles discuss the basic pathogenesis, keypoints for differentiation, main therapeutic rule and major formula of severe *Yangming* obstruction syndrome. The basic pathogenesis is interior heat and dry stool altogether obstructing *Qi* of the large intestine seriously, so marked by severe constipation, or occasional watery discharge out from the anus at the side of the hot-dry stools (*Re Jie Pang Liu* 热结旁流）, abdominal fullness and distention without diminution or no evident decrease, pain around the navel with tenderness, or dry stools palpated by hand, tidal fever intensified at 3~5 pm, sometimes delirium, thirst, fidgets, ceaseless sweating, hunger with over eating or failure to eat food, red tongue with yellow or black and prickle coating, and a slippery-rapid or a deep-unsmooth-forceful pulse.

Da Chengqi Tang has a strongest action in terms of both clearing away dryness-heat and lowering intestinal *Qi* by a heavy purgation due to *Houpo* and *Zhishi* in large doses combined with *Dahuang* and *Mangxiao*, and *Dahuang* decocted later having a stronger action of purgation. Therefore, it belongs to a drastic purgative in TCM and is used for severe *Yangming* obstruction syndrome. In addition, since the formula has a very strong purgative action, it must be used carefully and temporarily.

Da Chengqi Tang possesses strong pharmacological actions of both *Tiaowei Chengqi Tang* and *Xiao Chengqi Tang*, and its comprehensive therapeutic effects are stronger than the other two formulas. It can be applied for a lot of diseases in modern Western medicine, such as epidemic encephalitis B, acute hepatitis, pneumonia, appendicitis, nephritis, dysentary, intestinal obstruction, and so forth.

Comparison among the Syndromes of Three *Chengqi Tang*

Three *Chengqi Tang* syndromes	*Tiaowei Chengqi Tang* Syndrome	*Xiao Chengqi Tang* Syndrome	*Da Chengqi Tang* Syndrome
Pathogenesis	Early aggregation of excess heat with severe dryness-heat and less *Qi* stagnation	Middle degree of excess heat with severer *Qi* blockage and less dryness-heat	Most serious *Yangming* obstruction with equal dryness-heat and *Qi* blockage
Main manifestation	Steaming fever, much sweating, severe vexation and thirst, delirious speech, sore swollen and ulcerative throat	Abdominal distention, pain and tenderness, constipation or difficulty in defecation, frequent flatulence	Severe abdominal distention, fulless, pain and tenderness, constipation, tidal fever intensified in afternoon, Delirium or mania
Clinical characteristics	Marked dryness, heat and solidity; slight stuffiness, fullness and pain	Marked stuffiness, fullness and pain; slight dryness, heat, and solidity	Dryness, heat, hardness, fullness, distention and pain all are heavy

Article 220

In an amalgamation of *Taiyang* and *Yangming* patterns, if the *Taiyang* pattern has disappeared, and there are tidal fever, ceaseless sweating from the limbs, difficulty in defecation and delirious speech, catharsis will bring on recovery, and *Da Chengqi Tang* is appropriate.

Synopsis	The primary symptoms and treatment of severe *Yangming* obstruction syndrome transformed from an amalgamation syndrome.

Commentary	In this amalgamation syndrome, it is likely that *Taiyang* pattern appears first, then *Yangming* pattern follows. Presently, tidal fever, difficulty in defecation, delirium and ceaseless sweating on the limbs, all show there is a severe *Yangming* obstruction syndrome left after the *Taiyang* pattern has disappeared, so it can be treated by *Da Chengqi Tang*.

Application	The development direction of a concurrent occurred syndrome or an amalgamation syndrome depends upon all of the patient's manifestations at that moment present instead of the prior days that he experienced the disease and others according to this article, withtreatment treatment aiming at the present syndrome.

Article 242

A patient presenting dysuria, irregularly difficult or easy defecation, sometimes slight fever, dyspnea and vertigo with inability to lie flat, all indicate dry stool stagnation in the large intestine, so *Da Chengqi Tang* can be used for adequate treatment.

Article 212

A cold-induced disease unrelieved after emesis or catharsis, marked by no defecation for 5 or 6 days, even up to more than ten days, tidal fever at 3~5 in the afternoon, no aversion to cold, and soliloquy as if seeing ghosts. In the severe cases, there are an unconsciousness with picking at their clothing and bedclothes unreasonably, fright with disquiet, deficient dyspnea, and staring forward, which will be favorable in case of a wiry pulse, and unfavorable in case of an unsmooth pulse. The mild cases with fever and delirious speech, should be treated mainly by *Da Chengqi Tang*. Stop taking the rest of decoction if the patient has a defecation after taking the first dose.

Synopsis	The main symptoms, treatment and prognosis of dangerous *Yangming* obstruction syndrome.
Commentary	The syndomes in these two articles are more serious and dangerous. In Article 242, dysuria is caused by intense heat impairing body fluid, difficulty in defecation and slight fever by heat and dry stool obstructed in the large intestine; furthermore, easy defecation is due to a part of body fluid kept still in the intestine due to dysuria. The turbid pathogen (dry stool with heat and stagnant *Qi*) upwardly clouds the clear orifices, thus giveing rise to vertigo, and upward attacking the lung, thus leading to serious dyspnea with failure to lie flat, both signifying an urgent and dangerous situation, in which two important organs, i.e., the lung and brain, have been significantly impaired, and should be treated with *Da Chengqi Tang* in time.

Article 212 discusses a more critical condition based on the *Yangming* obstruction syndrome. Constipation for many days, tidal fever and delirium are main symptoms of severe *Yangming* obstruction syndrome, precisely treated by *Da Chengqi Tang*. However, unconsciousness, soliloquy（*Duyu* 独语）as if seeing ghosts, picking at their clothing and bedclothes unreasonably（*Xunyi Mochuang* 循衣摸床）and fright with disquiet all belong to serious mental disturbances, which result from simultaneous rampant pathogens and depletion of vital *Qi* in the body.

Meanwhile, deficient dyspnea here is caused by the kidney failing to hold *Qi* due to exhaustion of kidney-*Yin*, and staring forward by stirring up of liver-wind due to depletion of essence-blood of liver-kidney. All the above mentioned suggest an extremely serious syndrome marked by intense pathogen combined with exhausted vital *Qi*, and it may be favorable in case of a wiry-long pulse, which indicates that vital *Qi* can still struggle against the pathogen, but it may be unfavorable in case of an unsmooth-short pulse, which indicates that extreme heat has depleted *Yin* fluid.

Article 252

The cold-induced disease lasting for 6 or 7 days, marked by blurred vision, inability to move eyeballs agilely, with neither exterior syndrome nor an interior one, difficult defecation, and slight fever, which indicate an excess pattern; this should be treated by urgent catharsis, and *Da Chengqi Tang* is indicated.

Article 253

Yangming pattern marked with fever and profuse sweating, can be treated by urgent catharsis and *Da Chengqi Tang* is appropriate.

Article 254

The cold-induced disease unrelieved after diaphoresis, marked with abdominal fullness and pain, can be treated by urgent catharsis and *Da Chengqi Tang* is appropriate.

Synopsis　　Main symptoms and treatment of the three syndromes by urgent catharsis so as to preserve *Yin* fluid.

Commentary　　In *Yangming* obstruction syndrome, there are some specially urgent situations owing to intense heat depleting *Yin* seriously, so one must use *Da Chengqi Tang* to preserve *Yin* by urgent purgation.

First, sudden blurred vision with staring shows that violent dryness-heat consumes liver-*Yin*, then leading to internal stirring up of liver-wind; secondly, fever and profuse sweating both seriously exhaust *Yin* fluid; and thirdly, abdominal fullness and pain after diaphoresis suggest that exterior pathogen transformed into heat in the interior and lack of body fluid, both indicating a severe dryness-heat and *Yin* depletion. Therefore, these three serious situations need to be treated by urgent catharsis, such as *Da Chengqi Tang*, otherwise, the patient may be going to die due to progressive *Yin* exhaustion.

Application　　These three articles tell us that the *Yangming* pattern, especially *Yangming* obstruction syndrome easily develops into *Yin* exhaustion（*Wang Yin* 亡阴）, which should be treated urgently by *Da Chengqi Tang* if intense dryness-heat leads to *Yin* deficiency. Of course, the formula cannot be used if obstruction of internal heat and dry stool is mild or non-existent.

Article 247

A patient's *Fuyang* (on the instep) pulse is floating and unsmooth, where the floating pulse implies a hyperactivity of the stomach, the unsmooth pulse implies frequent urination, and both pulses together imply hardening of stool and formation of restrained spleen disorder, which should be treated mainly with *Maziren Wan*.

Maziren Wan	*Huomaren* 20 g, *Dahuang* 9 g, *Zhishi* 9 g, *Houpo* 9 g, *Baishao* 9 g, *Xingren* 9 g and *Fengmi* in proper amounts.
Synopsis	Main symptoms, pulse, pathogenesis and treatment of restrained spleen disorder.
Commentary	Restrained Spleen Disorder（*Piyue* 脾约）appears in a cold-induced disease and can be seen as a mild *Yangming* obstruction syndrome, caused by the stomach heat leading to a restraint on the spleen in the transportation of body fluid, namely, too much fluid flowing into the bladder and less fluid flowing into the large intestine, resulting in dry and hard stools, frequent urination, and a floating and unsmooth pulse on *Fuyang*, where the Foot-*Yangming* Meridian passes through, thus reflecting the functions of the spleen-stomach. The other symptoms may include dry mouth, restlessness, mild abdominal fullness and distention, and red-dark tongue with yellow-dry coating. All the manifestations indicate a deficiency of body fluid with mild dryness-heat in the gastrointestinal tract leading to *Qi* stagnation, and can be seen as a mild type of *Yangming* obstruction.
	Maziren Wan belongs to a slight purgative, because *Huomaren*, *Xingren*, *Baishao* and *Fengmi* together have a heavy action to moisten the large intestine to induce bowel movement; and contains the ingredients of *Xiao Chengqi Tang*, thus can lower *Qi* and clear heat by catharsis, and the preparation form of a pill makes its effect slower and moderate.
Application	Since *Maziren Wan* has a very slight and slow action for purgation, it is extensively applied for the treatment of various chronic types of constipation, especially habitual constipation, and constipation in old people and postpartum women, or during the restoration period after a febrile disease, paralytic ileus and other chronic diseases, which are all ascribable to lack of body fluid and mild dryness-heat in the gastrointestinal tract.

Article 204

A cold induced disease with frequent vomiting cannot be treated by catharsis even though it belongs to *Yangming* pattern.

Article 205

Yangming pattern marked with epigastric hardness and fullness cannot be treated by catharsis, because of ceaseless diarrhea after purgation, which implies an unfavorable prognosis, or may recover if the diarrhea stops spontaneously.

Article 206

Yangming pattern with flushing on the whole face can not be treated by catharsis. And a fever and yellowish skin must accompany with dysuria after purgation.

Article 189

Yangming pattern with exterior syndrome, marked by bitter taste in the mouth, dry throat, abdominal fullness, slight dyspnea, fever with aversion to cold, and a floating and tense pulse, there would be severer abdominal fullness and difficult urination after using a purgative.

Article 194

Yangming pattern with inability to eat food due to underlying deficiency-cold in the stomach, must result in a hiccup after using cathartic to clear away heat.

Synopsis	Five pathological conditions for catharsis all involving in the *Yangming* obstruction syndrome.
Commentary	These five articles discuss five types of pathlogical conditions that are unable to be treated by catharsis. Article 204 implies that a *Yangming* heat syndrome without a combination of dry stool in the intestine, along with adverse ascending of the stomach-heat leading to frequent vomiting. For this situation, catharsis cannot be used for the *Yangming* heat syndrome with an adverse ascent of *Qi*, because it is contrary to an important therapeutic principle, i.e., treating a disease along its trend of development.

Article 205 points out that *Yangming* heat syndrome marked by epigastric hardness and fullness suggest shapeless heat stagnating in the stomach instead of shaped pathogen combines with heat in the intestines like *Yangming* obstruction syndrome. Thus application of a purgative will damage *Qi* or *Yang* of the spleen-stomach, giving rise to ceaseless diarrhea.

Article 206 introduces a *Yangming* pattern with flushing on the whole face pertaining to *Yangming* heat syndrome, which can be treated by *Baihu Tang* instead of a cathartic. So, there would be a fever, *Yang* jaundice and dysuria due to damp-heat accumulation resulting from deficiency of spleen-stomach after purgation.

Article 189 discusses an actual concomitant occurrence of three *Yang* patterns. Here fever with aversion to cold and a floating-tense pulse belong to *Taiyang* pattern, bitter taste in the mouth and dry throat to *Shaoyang* pattern, and abdominal fullness and slight dyspnea without abdominal pain, tenderness and constipation to *Yangming* heat syndrome. However, these three syndromes usually are contraindications of catharsis, if they are treated by catharsis, the exterior pathogen is easily transformed into interior heat, and then further consumes *Qi* and body fluid, so manifested as severer abdominal fullness and difficult defecation.

Yangming obstuction syndrome with inability to eat food may be caused by the intestinal turbid pathogen fuming upward and then leading to disturbance of the stomach. However, *Yangming* pattern in Article 194 is different; it is due to defiency-cold in the stomach, so there would be hiccup resulting from further decline of *Yang Qi* of the spleen-stomach after inppropriate catharsis.

| Application | These five articles tell us that cold-natured purgatives like *Da Chengqi Tang* are only used for *Yangming* obstruction syndrome, and do not apply to *Yangming* heat syndrome, *Taiyang* or *Shaoyang* pattern, especially any deficiency-cold syndrome for that matter, which all should be observed by TCM doctors. |

Section 5 — Concomitant and Transmuted Syndromes of *Yangming* Pattern

Article 236

Yangming pattern with fever and sweating, suggests outward discharge of the heat pathogen, and thus no formation of jaundice. If there are sweating seen only on the head and neck, absence of sweating on other parts of the body, dysuria and thirst with intake of drinks, all indicate that the heat with damp stagnated in the interior and certainly producing jaundice, then this should be treated mainly by Yinchenhao Tang.

| Yinchenhao Tang | *Yinchen* 18 g, *Zhizi* 12 g and *Dahuang* 6 g. |

Decoct *Yinchen* with 1200 ml water first, and when the decoction is concentrated into 600 ml, put *Zhizi* and *Dahuang* into it and then decocted again, finally obtaining 300 ml decoction after removal of the dregs, and then is divided into three equal parts, and one part taken each time. The patient will have smooth urination with a brown-turbid color like solution of Chinese honey locust after taking the decoction, and abdominal fullness becomes relieved one night later, indicating that the jaundice was reduced following urination.

Article 260

A cold-induced disease lasting for 7 or 8 days, and marked by yellowish-bright skin like orange peel, dysuria and mild abdominal fullness-distention, should be treated mainly with *Yinchenhao Tang*.

Article 199

Yangming pattern accompanied by anhidrosis, dysuria, and dysphoria with oppressive chest will form jaundice.

| Synopsis | The formative mechanism, basic symptoms and treatment of the jaundice caused mainly by heat pathogen with damp stagnated in the interior. |

| Commentary | These three articles together discuss one of the concomitant syndromes of *Yangming* pattern, which can be seen as a result of internal heat with damp accumulating in the liver-gallbladder and spleen-stomach. *Yangming* pattern denotes an excess-heat syndrome in the interior, in which fever but no sweating is evident, or with sweating only above the neck, suggests heat with damp not being expelled from the body surface. Basically, dysuria suggests damp-heat unrelieved by urination, thus still accumulating in the middle *jiao* and leading further to *Qi* obstruction of the liver-gallbladder and reverse flow of bile into blood vessels, manifested as a *Yang*-jaundice. This presents with a bright-yellowish color like orange peel, thirst with desire for drinks, abdominal distention-fullness, loss of appetite, bitter taste in the mouth, dysphoria with oppressive chest, constipation or unsmooth defecation, red tongue with yellow-greasy |

coating, and a slippery or wiry-rapid pulse.

In *Yinchenhao Tang*, *Yinchen* removes damp-heat by diuresis to diminish jaundice first, while *Zhizi* and *Dahuang* both assist *Yinchen* in relieving jaundice by clearing heat to detoxify and inducing urination and purgation.

| Application | *Yinchenhao Tang* has been regarded as a basic and representative formula for a *Yang*-jaundice syndrome with heat predominant over damp. It has been found out in recent years that this formula has multiple effective actions, such as protecting liver, promotiong excretion of bile, lowering blood fat, reducing transaminase, abatement of fever, catharsis, diuresis, hemostasis, diminishing serum bilirubin, anti-mutation, relieving gastrointestinal spasms, anti-inflammation, anti-biosis, anti-virus, etc., and often applied in the treatment of severe hepatitis, infantile posthepatitis, hepatitis A, B, C, chronic hepatitis, hepatic injury due to chemotherapy or alcoholism, obesity, liver cirrhosis, liver cancer, acute or chronic cholecystitis, gallstones, seborrheic dermatitis, contact dermatitis, multiple stomatitis, acute conjunctivitis, lobar pneumonia, duodenal ulcer and appendicitis, all caused by pathogenic damp-heat accumulated in the interior with predominant heat. |

Article 261

A cold-induced disease marked by jaundice and fever, should be treated mainly by *Zhizi Baipi Tang*.

| *Zhizi Baipi Tang* | *Zhizi* 12 g, *Huangbai* 6 g and *Zhi Gancao* 3 g. |

| Synopsis | Main symptoms and treatment of a mild *Yang*-jaundice characterized with greater heat than damp. |

| Commentary | An exogenous disease is marked by fever and jaundice must be *Yang*-jaundice and present a bright-yellow color of the skin, eyes and urine like orange peel, dysphoria, thirst with excessive drinking, less or local |

sweating, scanty-hot urine, red tongue with yellow-dry coating, and a slippery-rapid pulse.

Comparing with *Yinchenhao Tang* syndrome, *Zhizi Baipi Tang* syndrome belongs to mild *Yang*-jaundice with evident heat and slight damp, and without obvious *Qi* obstruction of the gastrointestinal tract.

Application   *Zhizi Baipi Tang* may be used for a mild case of *Yang*-jaundice with less damp. So, it is often used in combination with other formulas for cases of *Yang*-jaundice when the disease is more serious and complicated.

Article 262

A cold-induced disease marked pathologically by stagnated heat-damp in the interior and certainly presenting jaundice, should be treated mainly with *Mahuang Lianqiao Chixiaodou Tang*.

Mahuang Lianqiao Chixiaodou Tang   *Mahuang* 6 g, *Lianqiao* 6 g, *Xingren* 9 g, *Chixiaodou* 20 g, *Sangbaipi* 20 g, *Shengjiang* 6 g, *Dazao* 9 g and *Zhi Gancao* 6 g.

Synopsis   Basic pathogenesis, symptoms and treatment of *Yang*-jaundice with a mild exterior syndrome in the early stage.

Commentary   The article introduces a syndrome of *Yang*-jaundice with a mild exterior syndrome in its early stage, based on inference from the formula used. *Yang*-jaundice means damp-heat pathogen accumulation in the interior, marked by gradually obvious bright-yellowish skin, eyes and urine, dysuria, bitter taste and dryness in the mouth, but drinking less, restlessness, loss of appetite, heavy body, red tongue with yellow-greasy coating and a soft-rapid pulse, thus *Lianqiao, Chixiaodou* and *Sangbaipi* are used.

However, *Mahuang, Shengjiang* and *Xingren* in the formula are used for a mild exterior syndrome, which presents as aversion to cold, fever, no sweating, headache, slight cough, and floating pulse. *Dazao* and *Gancao* normalize the spleen-stomach. Therefore, this syndrome can be treated effectively by this formula because of its action in removing damp-heat by diuresis and expelling pathogen outward from the exterior.

| Application | *Mahuang Lianqiao Chixiaodou Tang* possesses actions of anti-pyretogenesis, diuresis, detoxication, relieving cough and asthma, diaphoresis and anti-allergy, so it can be applied for such diseases in Western medicine as acute icteric hepatitis, acute nephritis, acute pyelonephritis, acute cholecystitis, allergic skin diseases, allergic rhinitis, conjunctivitis, urticaria, purpura, acute bronchitis and acute broncheal asthma. |

Article 237

Yangming syndrome with forgetfulness mostly caused by underlying blood stasis in a long time, marked by hard and black stools but that are easily defecated, is suitably treated with *Didang Tang* to purge downward.

Article 257

A patient has neither an exterior syndrome nor interior one, with fever lasting for 7 or 8 days, or constipation for 6 or 7 days and easy hunger, and if pulse is floating-rapid or still rapid after catharsis, it should be purgated with *Didang Tang*, because there is a combination of internal heat and blood stasis.

Didang Tang	Seeing section 4 of the chapter *Taiyang* pattern.
Synopsis	Basic pathogenesis, symptoms and treatment of *Yangming* blood-retention (*Yangming Xuxue* 阳明蓄血) syndrome.
Commentary	*Yangming* blood-retention syndrome has a basic pathogenesis, namely, internal heat and blood stasis agglomerating in the stomach and intestine,

arising from one of two ways, *Yangming* heat or obstruction syndrome combined with an underlying blood stasis in the gastrointestinal tract, or heat pathogen in *Qi* phase after inappropriate catharsis consuming body fluid in the large intestine and concentrating the blood into blood stasis in the intestinal collaterals. For the former, there are hard and black stools but easily defecated; while for the latter, there is a long constipation with very dry feces. Meanwhile, the other main manifestations of this syndrome are fever or tidal fever, easy hunger, abdominal hardness-fullness or pain with tenderness, forgetfullness, delirium or even mania, thirst, deep red tongue with ecchymosis and yellow coating, and a slippery-rapid or deep-unsmooth pulse.

Didang Tang has a strong action to eliminate blood stasis and interior heat by purgation, so it suitable for this syndrome.

Application

The blood-retention syndrome can appear in both *Taiyang* pattern and *Yangming* pattern, but share the same basic pathogenesis, i.e., blood stasis combined with internal heat in the interior, especially in the intestines. The difference is only that one syndrome coming from *Yangming* pattern with severe intestinal obstruction, another one coming from *Taiyang* pattern with mild exterior syndrome.

Questions for Review and Thinking

1. How do you understand the outline of *Yangming* pattern? What is the relation between it and its two principal syndromes?

2. What are main differences between *Yangming* heat syndrome and *Yangming* obstruction syndrome in terms of basic symptoms and therapeutic rules? Why?

3. Compare the syndromes treated by *Tiaowei Chengqi Tang, Xiao Chengqi Tang, Da Chengqi Tang* and *Maziren Wan* in pathogenesis, chief symptoms,

therapeutic rule and main prescription.

4. What are the contraindications of cold-purgatives? Why?

5. *Yinchenhao Tang, Zhizi Baipi Tang* and *Mahuang Lianqiao Chixiaodou Tang* all can be used for *Yang*-jaundice. How to distinguish them in their actions, pathogenesis and indications?

6. What are the main pathogenesis, symptoms, therapeutic rule and formula for *Yangming* blood-retention syndrome? How to distinguish it from *Taiyang* blood-retention syndrome?

Chapter III

Differentiation of Symptoms, Pulses and Treatment of *Shaoyang* Pattern

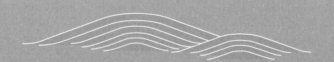

Article 263

In *Shaoyang* syndrome there must be bitter taste in the mouth, dry throat and blurred vision.

Synopsis

A part of the outline of *Shaoyang* pattern.

Commentary

Shaoyang pattern means the exogenous pathogen is wandering between the exterior and interior body, and then impeding the opening-closing movement of *Qi* of the body.

Meanwhile, Foot-*Shaoyang*, gallbladder, and Hand-*Shaoyang*, pericardium, both contain the minister fire. When an exogenous pathogen invades in *Shaoyang*, the gallbladder fails to keep a free flow of *Qi* and the stagnated minister fire transformed into fire pathogen. When the gallbladder-fire flames upward, the bile flows upward from the stomach into the mouth, resulting in bitter taste in the mouth; the fire damages the *Yin* fluid, resulting in dry throat; and the fire attacks upward into the eyes along with its meridians, thus blurred vision occurs.

However, this article cannot reflect the pathogenesis and main manifestations thoroughly, and according to the other articles in this chapter, *Shaoyang* pattern is caused comprehensively by the pathogen located in the half exterior and half interior, gallbladder fire attacking the spleen-stomach, and deficiency of stomach *Qi*. Therefore, it belongs actually to an excess mixed with deficiency syndrome.

Application

As an outline of *Shaoyang* pattern, this article is not complete, because it only points out a minority of the pathogenesis and symptoms, i.e., gallbladder-heat flaming upward and attacking the stomach and three symptoms they cause; however, it does not mention the other two basic pathogeneses and symptoms caused by both, such as the exogenous pathogen wandering between the exterior and interior, with *Qi* stagnation in the gallbladder, thus presenting alternate chills and fever, fullness in the hypochondrium and chest, mental depression, fidgeting, poor appetite, easy vomiting and wiry-thready pulse. So it is not sufficient for us to grasp the basic pathogenesis and primary manifestations limited in this article.

Article 97

When the blood is inadequate and *Qi* is weakened, the interstices of skin and muscles are often open, so the exogenous pathogen easily enters the body, struggles against the vital *Qi*, then the pathogen and stagnant *Qi* aggregate in the hypochondrium. The patient's predominant pathogen and vital *Qi* by turns leads to alternate chills and fever happening, and depressive silence with a loss of appetite due to hypofunction of spleen-stomach. Since the *Zang*-organs and *Fu*-organs are interconnected, if the gallbladder pathogen in the hypochondriac region intrudes into the spleen-stomach, it can give rise to hypochondriac and abdominal pain and vomiting. In this case, *Xiao Chaihu Tang* should be mainly adopted. If there is obvious thirst after taking this decoction, it indicates a transformation from *Shaoyang* pattern into *Yangming* one, and thus is treated accordingly as *Yangming* syndrome.

Synopsis	A supplementary to the pathogenesis, symptoms and treatment of *Shaoyang* pattern, and a possibility of *Shaoyang* pattern transformed into *Yangming* syndrome.

Commentary	This article can be divided into 4 paragraphs. The first paragraph points out that the patients suffering from *Shaoyang* pattern must entail a struggle between deficient vital *Qi* and a weak pathogen, consequently, the pathogen cannot invade deeply into the interior completely, and simultaneously, vital *Qi* cannot expel the pathogen out. Both wandering between the half exterior and half interior of the body, with *Qi* stagnation in the hypochondriac regions where *Shaoyang* meridians pass through, thus marked by alternate chills and fever, and hypochodriac ditention-fullness or even pain.

Secondly, when a stagnated gallbladder-heat attacks the stomach to induce its hypofunction and *Qi* stagnation, thus depressive silence with loss of appetite occurs.

Thirdly, the liver-gallbladder is located in the hypochondrium and superior to the spleen-stomach, if the pathogen of the gallbladder attacks the spleen-stomach, there would be abdominal pain and frequent vomiting. All of the 3 groups of symptoms are ascribed to a *Shaoyang* pattern and treated by *Xiao Chaihu Tang*.

Finally, if thirst gets worse after taking the decoction, it suggests that the *Shaoyang* pattern has been transformed into *Yangming* pattern, and requires treatment of *Yangming* syndrome.

Application   This article clearly emphasizes that the pathogen is wandering between the exterior and interior, and deficient *Qi* of spleen-stomach are the two main pathogenesis of *Shaoyang* pattern besides gallbladder-heat attacking the stomach mentioned in the above article. Usually, *Zhang Zhongjing* elaborated some symptoms often in terms of relative strength between vital *Qi* and pathogen, and pathological relations among the different *Zangfu*-organs, which have been used extensively to explain various manifestations in the later ages.

Why can the *Shaoyang* pattern transfer its pathogen into *Yangming* one? According to the *Neijing*, a typical type of transference should be from *Yangming* to *Shaoyang*, however, the transferring direction depends upon many factors, and the relative strength of vital *Qi* and pathogen is most important. For example, the *Taiyang* pattern may recover spontaneously in case of vital *Qi* overcoming the pathogen; it may transfer into three *Yin* patterns in case of the pathogen overcoming vital *Qi*; it may transfer into *Yangming* in case of both being strong; and it may transfer into *Shaoyang* in case of both being deficient. A *Shaoyang* pattern transfers its pathogen into *Yangming* in this article, it may be due to the patient's vital *Qi* and the heat patogen both becoming stronger.

Article 264

Shaoyang pattern with wind invasion, chracterized by sudden deafness, congested eyes, full chest and restlessness, cannot be treated by emesis and purgation, otherwise, palpitations and frightening may occur.

Article 265

A cold-induced disorder with headache, fever and wiry- thready pulse belong to *Shaoyang* pattern, and cannot be treated by diaphoresis, otherwise it may lead to delirious speech, indicating transformed *Yangming* obstruction syndrome marked with fidgeting and palpitations, which can be relieved by purgation to normalize the stomach.

Synopsis

A part of symptoms and contraindications of *Shaoyang* pattern and its an example of transmuted synsromes after wrong diaphoresis.

Commentary

These two articles give *Shaoyang* pattern more complements. Here, deafness and congested eyes show a flaming upward of the gallbladder-heat; full chest and restlessness implies the gallbladder-heat obstructing *Qi* flow in the chest and then disturbing the mind; headache, fever and a wiry-thready pulse together suggest an upward disturbance of gallbladder-fire with neither exterior syndrome nor intense interior heat syndrome, so it can be seen as a *Shaoyang* syndrome.

Shaoyang pattern does not belong to exterior syndrome, thus cannot be treated by diaphoresis, which may lead to delirium due to intensified internal heat. It is not located in the upper *Jiao* and lower *Jiao*, and no shaped pathogen in the interior, so emesis and purgation are not suitable for it. When such wrong treatments are used, palpitations, fright and fidgeting may happen due to deficiency of *Qi*-blood or aggravation of internal heat.

Application

Since *Shaoyang* pattern has a complicated pathogenesis, namely, combination of exterior and interior, heat and cold, excess and deficiency, so it can be treated only by harmonization instead of diaphoresis, emesis, purgation and pure tonification.

Section 2   Differentiation and Treatment of *Shaoyang* Pattern

Article 96

A cold-induced disease with wind invasion lasting for 5 or 6 days, marked by alternate chills and fever, fullness and distention in the chest and hypochondrium, depressive silence with loss of appetite, dysphoria and frequent vomiting, or oppressive sensation in the chest without vomiting, or thirst, or abdominal pain, or hypochondriac stuffiness-hardness, or palpitation and dysuria, or absence of thirst with a slight fever, or cough, should be treated mainly with *Xiao Chaihu Tang*.

Xiao Chaihu Tang   *Chaihu* 24 g, *Huangqin* 9 g, *Banxia* 12 g, *Shengjiang* 9 g, *Renshen* 9 g, *Dazao* 9 g and *Zhi Gancao* 9 g.

Decoct the above 7 drugs with cold water 1200 ml, and remove the dregs after the decoction reduced into 600 ml, then decoct it continuously until the decoction concentrated into 300 ml, which is then divided into 3 equal portions. Each portion taken orally each time, 3 times a day. In case of an oppressive chest without vomiting, remove *Banxia* and *Renshen*, add *Gualou* 15 g; in case of thirst, remove *Banxia* and add *Renshen* up to 14 g and *Tianhuafen* 12 g; in case of abdominal pain, remove *Huangqin* and add *Baishao* 9 g; in case of hypochondriac stuffiness-hardness, remove *Dazao* and add Muli 12 g; in case of palpitations and dysuria, remove *Huangqin* and add *Fuling* 12 g; in case of low fever on the exterior without thirst, remove *Renshen* and add *Guizhi* 9 g, awaiting a recovery following slight sweating after taking the decoction and covered with a quilt; moreover, in case of cough, remove *Renshen*, *Dazao* and *Shengjiang*, then add *Wuweizi* 12 g and *Ganjiang* 6 g.

Synopsis	Main symptoms and treatment of *Shaoyang* pattern.

Commentary	*Taiyang* pattern lasting for 5 or 6 days unrelieved indicates neither vital *Qi* overcoming pathogen nor pathogen overcoming vital *Qi*, both struggling and wandering between the exterior and interior, thus manifested as alternate chills and fever; the meridian *Qi* of *Shaoyang* is obstructed by the pathogen, and gallbladder *Qi* fails to flow freely, so there is fullness-distention in the chest and hypochondrium; *Qi* stagnation of the liver and gallbladder and further attacking of the spleen-stomach, resulting in depressive silence with loss of appetite; furthermore, the gallbladder fire transformed from the exterior pathogen is then disturbing the mind and over-restraining the stomach, leading to an adverse ascending of stomach *Qi*, so dysphoria with frequent vomiting happens. These 4 smptoms plus a bitter taste in the mouth, dry throat and blurred vision in Article 263 are seen as the 7 basic symptoms of *Shaoyang* pattern, all caused mainly by a complicated pathogenesis, i.e., firstly, an exogenous pathogen wandering in the half-exterior and half-interior; secondly, the gallbladder fire attacking the spleen-stomach, and thirdly, deficiency and an adverse ascent of stomach *Qi*.

Therefore, *Shaoyang* pattern belongs to heat mixed with cold syndrome, excess with deficiency syndrome, and concurrent existence of the exterior and interior syndromes. The other symptoms behind "or" in the original text are all possibly concomitant manifestations of *Shaoyang* pattern and are not always present.

Xiao Caihu Tang is a major formula for *Shaoyang* pattern and also the most basic prescription in *Shanghan Lun*. In the formula, *Chaihu* disperses pathogen outward in the half-exterior, *Huangqin* clears away heat in the half-interior, both together harmonize *Shaoyang* and activate gallbladder-*Qi*; *Banxia* and *Shengjiang* invigorate the spleen and lower *Qi* to normalize stomach and stop vomiting; *Renshen, Dazao* and *Gancao* regulate spleen-stomach and support vital *Qi* to eliminate the pathogen. The specific preparation of the formula is to concentrate its effective components and moderate its therapeutic action. The oppressive chest without vomiting suggests phlegm and heat accumulating in the chest, thus *Renshen* and *Banxia* must be removed due to their warm or/and greasy nature, and *Gualou* must be added to dispel phlegm-heat and ease the chest. Thirst here suggests gallbladder fire damaging body fluid, so removing the warm-dry *Banxia* is necessary to avoid impairing *Yin*; adding *Renshen* and *Tianhuafen* to produce body fluid and clear heat. Abdominal pain denotes gallbladder pathogen over-restraining the spleen, so *Huangqin* must be removed because of its bitter-cold nature further impairing the spleen; finally, adding *Baishao* to relieve pain by relaxing the tendons. Hypochondriac stuffiness-hardness is due to *Qi* stagnation of *Shaoyang*, leading to agglomeration of fluid-retention in the hypochondriac region, thus sweet and greasy *Dazao* must be removed, and adding *Muli* to dissolve fluid-retention and soften hardness to diminish the agglomeration. Palpitations and dysuria together are caused by fluid-retention in the interior due to *Yang* deficiency, thus getting rid of the bitter-cold natured *Huangqin* and adding *Fuling* is necessary to expel fluid-retention by inducing diuresis. Absence of thirst with slight fever indicates the interior heat sparing body fluid and still presentng a mild exterior syndrome, thus getting rid of greasy *Renshen* is necessary to avoid retaining the pathogen and adding *Guizhi* to relieve the exterior syndrome by expelling wind. Here cough results from cold fluid-retention in the lung, so sweet and greasy *Renshen* and *Dazao* must be removed, along with *Shengjian* due to its strong outward scattered action impairing *Yang Qi*; add *Ganjiang* to warm the lung for dissolving fluid-retention, and add *Wuweizi* to stop cough by astringing the lung *Qi*.

| Application | *Xiao Chaihu Tang* has multiple therapeutic functions, such as relieving fever, anti-inflammation, promoting bile excretion, reducing vomiting and relieving pain, so it has been extensively applied over decades for common cold, influenza, headache, abdominal pain, jaundice, hypochondriac pain, vertigo, postpartum fever, tinnitus, deafness, etc. *Chaihu* requires a large dosage when used for a high fever. |

Article 266

Taiyang pattern has not relieved and then transformed into Shaoyang pattern, manifested as hypochondriac hardness and fullness, retching with inability to eat, alternate chills and fever, and deep-tense pulse, can be treated by Xiao Chaihu Tang, if it hasn't been treated by emesis and purgation.

Synopsis

Main manifestations and treatment of *Shaoyang* pattern transformed just from *Taiyang* pattern before long.

Commentary

Shaoyang pattern can be formed from either direct invasion into *Shaoyang Fu*-organ and the meridian by an exogenous pathogen, or transformation from *Taiyang* pattern if the patient's vital *Qi* and pathogen are both not strong enough. Here, *Qi* stagnation of the gallbladder organ and its meridian can cause hypochondriac hardness and fullness, stagnated gallbladder-heat attacking the stomach transversely leads to retching with inability to eat, and predominance of both, in turn, gives rise to the alternate chills and fever. These three symptoms can be regarded as the most important and significant clinical manifestations for differentiation of the *Shaoyang* pattern.

The syndrome in this article comes from *Taiyang* pattern, but now there are three main symptoms of *Shaoyang* pattern and no symptom of *Taiyang* pattern, implying that it has completed a transformation, then *Xiao Chaihu Tang* can be used. Here, a deep pulse just indicates the pathogen deeply invades from the exterior, and a tense pulse is similar to wiry pulse. Both pulses in Eastern *Han* Dynasty were not standarized yet, thus having a similar clinical significance.

Application

Xiao Chaihu Tang is a basic formula of *Shaoyang* pattern, but it can be used in different syndromes resulting from the multiple causes and based on various main symptoms. This article shows that it can be used for a transmuted syndrome from *Taiyang* pattern even if the case has only a part of *Shaoyang* symptoms without a typical pulse.

Article 101

Either the cold or wind invasion syndrome has been transformed into *Chaihu Tang* syndrome, which can be confirmed according to only one main symptom, so it is unnecessary for a doctor to await all the symptoms to appear simultaneously. When the *Xiao Chaihu Tang* syndrome is treated by catharsis only, if the syndrome has not disappeared, this formula can be given again, and it will be relieved after a fever and sweating; this follows a steamed feeling and shivery limbs.

Synopsis

An important principle for flexibly applying *Xiao Chaihu Tang* and the effective signs of administration of *Xiao Chaihu Tang* after misuse of catharsis.

Commentary

Shaoyang pattern, also called *Xiao Chaihu Tang* syndrome, should be treated mainly by *Xiao Chaihu Tang*, however, the clinical application of this formula is very flexible, because *Shaoyang* pattern has a very complicated pathogenesis, concretely, it is an easily changed syndrome in the transient stage of an exogenous disease, and often has diverse, indefinite, non-typical and incomplete symptoms, hence why *Xiao Chaihu Tang* syndrome "can be confirmed according to only one main symptom". Here, "main symptom" refers to one of the basic symptoms of *Shaoyang* pattern, which can reflect the three main pathogeneses mentioned before, including alternate chills and fever, fullness-distention in the chest and hypochondrium, depressive silence with loss of appetite, dysphoria with frequent vomiting or retching, bitter taste in the mouth, dry throat, blurred vision, and a wiry-thready pulse, so *Xiao Chaihu Tang* can be used flexibly, optionally and extensively for a lot of disorders; this applies only if they include one or a part of the main symptoms of *Shaoyang* pattern and are consistent with one of the three pathogeneses.

The second part of this article also reflects that *Shaoyang* pattern, after a wrong catharsis, can be still treated by *Xiao Chaihu Tang* only if the main symptoms of *Shaoyang* pattern still exist, because wrong purgation must further injure vital *Qi* and benifit the pathogen, and this formula can support vital *Qi* and expel pathogen at the same time. When an acute struggle between both gives rise to a steamed feeling with shivery body, and then the fever relieved following much sweating, which has been known as "shivering sweating" (*Zhanhan* 战汗) in later dynasties, and have a favorable prognosis as fever gradually relieves and the pulse becomes moderate after mild sweating.

Application

Since *Xiao Chaihu Tang* has very diverse and flexible therapeutic functions, its modifications have been used for a variety of diseases and symptoms, only if one or two main symptoms suggest a link to one or two main pathogeneses really exsisting, no matter whether *Xiao Chaihu Tang* syndrome is complete or not.

The term "shivering sweating" has been extensively quoted in the later ages, especially by the specialists of warm disease in the *Qing* Dynasty. This condition is considered as a turning point in the course of some acute exogenous or febrile diseases due to a fierce struggle between vital *Qi* and pathogen in the patient, and include two opposite prognoses: either the patient will gradually recover if his vital *Qi* overcomes the pathogen, manifesting as fever relief, restless mentality becoming quiet and hurried-rapid pulse changed into a calm one, or his diseased state will be deteriorating if the pathogen overcomes vital *Qi*.

Article 230

Yangming pattern marked by hypochondriac hardness-fullness, constipation, vomiting and white tongue coating, may give Xiao Chaihu Tang. And then all symptoms may be relieved with an unceasingly general sweating due to Qi of the upper Jiao restoring a smooth flow, thus the body fluid distributes downward and the stomach functions normally.

Synopsis

Main manifestations, treatment and curative mechanism of *Shaoyang* pattern mixed with *Yangming* pattern.

Commentary

Yangming pattern marked by constipation seems to be *Yangming* obstruction syndrome, however, hardness-fullness in the hypochondrium instead of the abdomen, and white tongue coating instead of yellow-dry one, both suggest that *Shaoyang* pattern is the first and *Yangming* pattern is second in such a concomitant syndrome. Subsequently, *Xiao Chaihu Tang* can be used for it, because it is a major formula indicated for *Shaoyang* pattern, which can harmonize *Shaoyang* syndrome, namely, dispersing *Qi* of liver-gallbladder unobstructively in the chest, then distributing body fluid downward, and finally normalizing the functions of spleen-stomach in the middle *Jiao*, therefore, *Qi* and body fluid of the entire *Sanjiao* move smoothly, verified by unceasingly general sweating; afterwards, all the symptoms of both *Shaoyang* and *Yangming* syndromes are relieved.

This article also points out an available sign of *Xiao Chaihu Tang* achieving an effective result, i.e., a mild, unceasing sweating in the whole body, which indicates a smooth flow of *Qi* and body fluid, appearing after using this formula.

| Application | *Xiao Chaihu Tang* is applied in such a concomitant syndrome because not only is *Shaoyang* pattern more serious in it, but also the formula can harmonize the exterior and interior, and promote *Qi* and body fluid in the whole body. |

Meanwhile, the description of the patient's reaction cured by *Xiao Chaihu Tang* can be seen as an obvious evidence of the *Shaoyang* pattern's basic pathogenesis and the formula's actions mentioned above.

—— **Article 229** ————

***Yangming* pattern with tidal fever, loose stool, smooth urination, and persistent fullness-distention in the chest and hypochondrium, *Xiao Chaihu Tang* may be given.**

| Synopsis | Main symptoms and treatment of *Shaoyang* pattern with *Yangming* pattern. |

| Commentary | Here "*Yangming* pattern" denotes there is an internal excess-heat syndrome in it, but "tidal fever, loose stool, smooth urination" signify that internal heat is not serious and intestinal obstruction syndrome hasn't developed. |

Meanwhile, persistent distention in the chest and hypochondriac region suggests there is a longer and severer *Shaoyang* pattern, so this case belongs to a concurrent occurrence of *Shaoyang* and *Yangming* patterns whereby the *Shaoyang* pattern is more serious, and *Xiao Chaihu Tang* can be used.

| Application | The above two articles show that *Xiao Chaihu Tang* is selected first for a concurrent occurrence of *Shaoyang* pattern with *Yangming* pattern. This is because the formula can harmonize both the exterior and interior, besides clearing heat and tonifying vital *Qi*, thus avoiding the side effect of the basic formulas for *Yangming* patterns, such as damaging spleen-stomach dut to excessive bitter-cold nature of *Baihu Tang* and *Chengqi Tang*. |

Article 99

Encountering cold-induced disorder for 4 or 5 days, manifested as fever, aversion to wind, stiff neck, hypochondriac fullness, warm extremities and thirst, should be mainly treated by *Xiao Chaihu Tang*.

| Synopsis | Main symptoms of concurrent occurrence of three *Yang* patterns treated basically by *Xiao Chaihu Tang*. |

| Commentary | "Cold-induced disorder for 4 or 5 days", denotes the exogenous pathogen from the exterior entering interior; the fever indicates that it still stays in the stage of *Yang* pattern according to *Neijing*, aversion to wind and stiff neck pertain to the *Taiyang* pattern, warm extrimities and thirst to the *Yangming* one, and hypochondriac fullness to the *Shaoyang* one, thus now becoming concurrent occurrence of three *Yang* patterns. Since *Taiyang* is located in the exterior body and tends to open, *Yangming* is in the interior and tends to close, while *Shaoyang* is in the middle and to pivot between the exterior and interior; *Xiao Chaihu Tang* can be chosen for treating this complex syndrome. |

| Application | *Xiao Chaihu Tang* is not only a formula for *Shaoyang* pattern, but can also be used for concurrent occurrence of two or three *Yang* patterns when the |

Shaoyang one is more serious. Of course, when the exterior syndrome or interior excess-heat is more obvious, the basic formulas of *Taiyang* or *Yangming* patterns are chosen first. However, *Xiao Chaihu Tang* is applied more frequently for concurrent occurrence and amalgamation of two or three *Yang* patterns because of its multiple and gentle actions.

—— Article 100

Cold-induced disorder marked by an unsmooth pulse on the right side and a wiry pulse on the left side, usually presenting with spasmodic pain in the abdomen, requires *Xiao Jianzhong Tang* first, then give *Xiao Chaihu Tang* next in case of no improvement.

Synopsis	Treatment of abdominal pain due to the pathogen of liver-galbladder attacking spleen-stomach.

Commentary

A spasmodic pain in the abdomen may have different pathogeneses. However, in this article, unsmooth pulse on the right *Cunkou* indicates *Qi* weakness of the spleen-stomach leading to deficiency of *Qi* and blood, and a wiry pulse on the left *Cunkou* denotes over-restraint of the liver-gallbladder onto the spleen-stomach, which is too weak. Therefore, first choosing *Xiao Jianzhong Tang* to treat *Ben* disorder, i.e., deficiency of *Qi* and blood, and secondarily using *Xiao Chaihu Tang* to treat *Biao* disorder, i.e., the liver-gallbladder over-restraining the spleen-stomach.

Application

The article tells us that although *Xiao Chaihu Tang* is a main formula for *Shaoyang* pattern in exogenous diseases, it can also be used for a lot of other diseases, such as headache, vomiting, epigastric stuffiness, hypochondriac pain, abdominal pain, diarrhea, malaria, irregular menstruation, mental depression, and protracted common cold with deficiency; only if patient's pathogeneses correspond to that of *Xiao Chaihu Tang*.

Next, TCM treatment should be consistent to the principle of *Biao-Ben*. Treating *Ben* first in the common cases, like that which article mentions; then, treating *Biao* first if *Biao* is urgent or very serious.

Concomitant and Transmuted Syndromes of *Shaoyang* Pattern

—— Article 267 ——

Delirium without *Xiao Chaihu Tang* syndrome after inducing vomiting, sweating, purgation or using warm-acupuncture, is known as deteriorated syndrome, should be treated by aiming at its pathogenesis based on the specific symptoms.

Synnopsis	The etiology and treatment principle of deteriorated syndrome of *Shaoyang* pattern.
Commentary	*Shaoyang* pattern should be treated by harmonization and *Xiao Chaihu Tang,* since emesis, diaphoresis, catharsis, and warm-acupuncture are all considered wrong therapies, as they may cause serious and dangerous disorders known as deteriorated syndromes, which include delirium, convulsion, high fever, hemorrhage, and dense skin eruption. The correct therapeutic principle for them is aiming at their concrete pathogeneses, obtained by analyzing all clinical manifestations, especially main presenting symptoms.
Application	This article like Article 16, in Section 5 of Chapter I talks about a fundamental principle for treatment of transmuted syndromes of all the six patterns; however, it is also considered as a sprout and core idea of TCM diagnosis and treatment, namely, *Bianzheng Shizhi.*

Article 146

The cold-induced exogenous disease lasting for 6 or 7 days, marked by fever with slight aversion to cold, vexing pain in the limb-joints, mild vomiting, epigastric stuffiness-hardness, and with existence of the exterior syndrome, should be treated mainly by _Chaihu Guizhi Tang_.

Chaihu Guizhi Tang	*Chaihu* 12 g, *Huangqin* 5 g, *Banxia* 6 g, *Renshen* 5 g, *Shengjiang* 5 g, *Dazao* 5 g, *Zhig Gancao* 3 g, *Guizhi* 5 g and *Baishao* 5 g.
Synopsis	The basic symptoms and treatment of concomitent Syndrome of *Shaoyang* pattern and *Taiyang* pattern.
Commentary	The exogenous disease lasting for 6 or 7 days should enter the interior body, but "fever with slight aversion to cold" and "vexing pain in the limb-joints" indicate *Taiyang* pattern with existent exterior syndrome; moreover, "mild vomiting" and "epigastric stuffiness-hardness" suggest that the gallbladder pathogen is attacking the stomach, so this is a concomitent syndrome of equally serious *Taiyang* and *Shaoyang* patterns. However, both are not typical and serious; consequently, both *Guizhi Tang* and *Xiao Chaihu Tang* in combination with their half dosages, known as *Chaihu Guizhi Tang*, can be used for this syndrome by relieving the exterior syndrome and harmonizing *Shaoyang* syndrome simultaneously.
Application	*Chaihu Guizhi Tang* belongs to the prescrition for relieving syndromes of both *Taiyang* and *Shaoyang* patterns, i.e., coordinating nutritive *Qi* and defensive *Qi* to expel the exterior pathogen and harmonizing between the gallbladder and stomach simultaneously, so it is often applied for common cold, influenza, pleuritis, gastric ulcer, duodenal bulbar ulcer, epilepsy, hysteria and neurosis in Western medicine, marked by the pathog enesis mentioned-above.

Article 103

Shaoyang pattern transformed from *Taiyang* syndrome for 10 or more days, is treated wrongly with catharsis 2 or 3 times, along with *Shaoyang* syndrome still existing after 4 or 5 days, *Xiao Chaihu Tang* should be given first. If the patient has incessant vomiting, epigastric contracted pain, and slightly depressive dysphoria, these indicate that the syndrome has not been relieved yet, so *Da Chaihu Tang* should be given to purge and then the syndrome will recover.

Da Chaihu Tang	*Chaihu* 24 g, *Huangqin* 9 g, *Banxia* 12 g, *Shengjiang* 15 g, *Dazao* 6 g, *Baishao* 9 g, *Zhishi* 12 g and *Dahuang* 6 g

Article 165

Cold-induced disease with fever unrelieved after sweating, meanwhile, with stuffiness-hardness in the chest and epigastrium, vomiting and diarrhea, should be treated mainly by *Da Chaihu Tang*.

Synopsis	The basic pathogenesis, symptoms and treatment of *Shaoyang* pattern with *Yangming* obstruction syndrome.

Commentary	*Shaoyang* pattern may be combined with *Yangming* obstruction syndrome after wrong treatment, e.g., frequent catharsis leading to the gallbladder heat pathogen invading into the gastrointestinal tract, followed by *Qi* obstruction in the *Fu*-organs, so marked by stuffiness-hardness or even contracted pain in the epigastric regions and abdomen with tenderness, thirst, fever unrelieved after sweating, and constipation or diarrhea with unsmooth defecation. At the same time, there is still the presence of *Shaoyang* symptoms, such as alternate chills and fever, hypochondriac distending pain, unceasing vomiting, depressive dysphoria, and bitter taste in the mouth. Therefore, *Da Chaihu Tang* is suitable for it. Of course, after wrong purgation, some cases yield only *Shaoyang* syndrome without symptoms of *Yangming* syndrome, *Xiao Chaihu Tang* can still be used.

Da Chaihu Tang is *Xiao Chaihu Tang* minus *Renshen* and *Gancao*, in combination with *Xiao Chengqi Tang* minus *Houpo* and plus *Baishao*, so it has two therapeutic actions, harmonizing *Shaoyang* and eliminating intestinal dryness-heat by purgation, thus it has been seen as a basic formula for concomitent syndrome of *Shaoyang* pattern and *Yangming* obstruction one.

Application	*Da Chaihu Tang* has many effective therapeutic actions in soothing *Qi* of the liver-gallbladder, promoting bile excretion, anti-inflmmation with relieving fever, inducing bowel movement, reducing sphincterismus, and removing toxins from the anus, etc. Therefore, it has been extensively applied for treatment of acute and chronic pancreatitis, cholecystitis, hepatitis, influenza, gallstone, acute perforation of peptic ulcer, peritonitis and so on.

Article 147

Cold-induced exogenous disease lasting 5 or 6 days after diaphoresis followed by catharsis, marked by fullness with slight hardness in the chest and hypochondrium, dysuria, thirst without vomiting, sweating only above the neck, alternate chills and fever, and dysphoria, all indicate that the disease has not been relieved yet, and should be treated mainly by *Chaihu Guizhi Ganjiang Tang*.

Chaihu Guizhi Ganjiang Tang	*Chaihu* 12 g, *Guizhi* 9 g, *Ganjiang* 6 g, *Tianhuafen* 12 g, *Huangqin* 9 g, Muli 9 g and *Zhi Gancao* 6 g
Synopsis	The basic pathogenesis, symptoms and treatment of *Shaoyang* syndrome with fluid-retention in the interior.
Commentary	The cold induced disease lasted 5 or 6 days after diaphoresis and then wrong catharsis is transformed from *Taiyang* pattern into a *Shaoyang* pattern, and meanwhile is combined with fluid-retention in the interior due to *Yang* damage. In this article, alternate chills and fever, fullness-stuffiness in the chest and hypochondrium, and dysphoria denote *Shaoyang*

syndrome, while dysuria, slight hardness in the chest and hypochondrium, thirst without vomiting and sweating above the neck are ascribed to fluid-retention with *Qi* stagnation in the chest-hypochondrium and *Sanjiao*, which is due to *Yang* deficiency in the middle *Jiao*.

Chaihu Guizhi Ganjiang Tang can be regarded as *Xiao Chaihu Tang* minus *Banxia*, *Shengjiang*, *Renshen* and *Dazao* because of fluid-retention in the interior except the stomach, and with *Guizhi* and *Ganjiang* added to warm *Yang* to dissolve fluid-retention, along with *Tianhuafen* and *Muli* to remove fluid-retention to soften hardness. So this formula can harmonize *Shaoyang* and dispel fluid-retention; furthermore, it warms *Yang* to invigorate the spleen and eliminate cold and heat pathogens concurrently.

Application	*Chaihu Guizhi Ganjiang Tang* has been used for many disorders such as common cold, cough, chest Bi, hypochondriac pain, epigastric pain, breast tumor and irregular menstruation in the later ages, only if they are caused by stagnation of gallbladder heat and fluid-retention in the interior. Based on the recent clinical reports, the modified formula can be applied for treatment of bronchitis, pneumonia, pleuritis, cholecystitis, chronic hepatitis, hyperplasia of mammary glands, and puerperal fever in Western medicine.

Article 107

Cold-induced exogenous disease lasting 8 or 9 days, then treated wrongly by catharsis, is characterized with fullness in the chest and hypochondrium, fidgets with fright-palpitations, dysuria, delirium, and a heavy feeling in the entire body with inability to turn sides to sides, should be treated mainly by *Chaihu Jia Longgu Muli Tang*.

Chaihu Jia Longgu Muli Tang	*Chaihu* 12 g, *Huangqin* 5 g, *Banxia* 5 g, *Renshen* 5 g, *Shengjiang* 5 g, *Dazao* 5 g, *Longgu* 9 g, *Muli* 9 g, *Qiandan* 5 g, *Dahuang* 6 g, *Guizhi* 5 g and *Fuling* 5 g.
Synopsis	The symptoms and treatment of *Shaoyang* pattern with heat and phlegm disturbing the mind after wrong treatment.

Lingering *Taiyang* pattern treated wrongly by catharsis brings about deep invasion of heat pathogen into the gallbladder and heart and with *Qi* deficiency, which gives rise to further endogenous production of phlegm-damp. The heat-phlegm of the gallbladder and heart obstructs *Qi* flow, presenting fullness in the chest and hypochondrium; disturbs the mind, manifesting as fidgets, frightful palpitations and even delirium; moreover, phlegm-damp resulting from *Qi* deficiency retains in the *Sanjiao* and the exterior body, presenting dysuria, a heavy body and inability to turn sides to sides. The other manifestations of this syndrome include bitter taste and dryness in the mouth, vertigo, headache, insomnia, irritability or even mania, red tongue with yellow-greasy coating, and a wiry-thready-rapid pulse.

Chaihu jia Longgu Muli Tang can be seen as *Xiao Chaihu Tang* minus *Gancao* and plus *Longgu, Muli, Qiandan, Dahuang, Guizhi* and *Fuling*, in which, *Chaihu* and *Huangqin* expel the pathogen from the gallbladder and interior, *Banxia, Shengjiang* and *Guizhi* warm the *Yang to* dissolve phlegm-damp and open the orifices, *Longgu, Muli* and *Qiandan* (a kind of toxic mineral drug, now replaced by *Cishi* or *Zheshi*) suppress the heart to calm the mind, *Dahuang* and *Fuling* remove heat and phlegm through defecation and urination respectively, while *Renshen* and *Dazao* strengthen *Qi*-blood of the heart and spleen to tranquilize. Therefore, this is an effective and complicated formula to harmonize *Shaoyang*, eliminate heat and phlegm-damp, and tonify vital *Qi* for tranquilization.

Chaihu Jia Longgu Muli Tang can be applied to treat a lot of mental diseases in Western medicine, such as schizophrenia, epilepsy, neurosis, Meniere's disease, heart diseases and hypertension as long as their pathogenesis share the same as that of this formula.

Article 172

For concurrent occurrence of both *Taiyang* and *Shaoyang* patterns marked chiefly by diarrhea, *Huangqin Tang* can be given; if it is associated with vomiting, *Huangqin Jia Banxia Shengjiang Tang* should be mainly given.

Huangqin Tang	*Huangqin* 9 g, *Baishao* 6 g, *Zhi Gancao* 6 g and *Dazao* 6 g.
Huangqin Jia Banxia Shengjiang Tang	above formula added with *Banxia* 12 g and *Shengjiang* 9 g.
Synopsis	Treatment of the diarrhea and vomiting in concurrent occurrence of *Taiyang* and *Shaoyang* patterns.

Commentary

This syndrome is actually marked by stagnated fire of *Shaoyang* invading into the stomach and intestine although it is said that *Taiyang* and *Shaoyang* patterns appear simultaneously; in other words, the pathological stress of this syndrome lies in the gallbladder fire attacking the gastrointestinal tract, which is one of the three pathogenesis of *Shaoyang* pattern, manifested as an acute diarrhea with yellow, watery and foul stool, hot feeling in the anus and unsmooth defecation, bitter taste and dryness in the mouth, abdominal pain, tenesmus, fever, restlessness, red tongue with yellow-dry coating, and a wiry-rapid pulse. It must be pointed out that the other basic symptoms of *Taiyang* and *Shaoyang* patterns exist but are not obvious, and the chief symptom in the former article is diarrhea, and the latter one is vomiting.

The syndrome takes gastrointestinal symptoms as the main manifestation, but the pathogen comes from *Shaoyang*, so *Huangqin* is used to clear away the stagnated fire of *Shaoyang*, while *Baishao* helps *Huangqin* to clear heat and relieve pain by relaxing the tendons; and *Gancao* and *Dazao* complement *Qi* to normalize spleen-stomach and coordinate *Baishao* to relieve pain. If the patient has severe vomiting, *Banxia* and *Shengjiang* are added to lower stomach *Qi* and thus stop vomiting.

Application

Huangqin Tang is used for not only heat natured diarrhea, but also dysentery and Spring warm disease in the later ages. For example, the famous prescription to treat dysentery, *Shaoyao Tang*, originated from this formula. At present, it is applied extensively for many diseases in Western medicine, such as acute and chronic gastritis and enteritis, bacterial dysentery, amebic dysentery, cholecystitis, neurogenic vomiting and so on.

Contrast between *Huangqin Tang* and *Gegen Qin Lian Tang*

Formula	*Huangqin Tang*	*Gegen Qin Lian Tang*
Basic Pathogenesis	Stagnated the gallbladder-heat attacking the large intestine.	Severe heat with mild damp invasion in the large intestine
Treatment	Clearing away heat to relieve diarrhea; next relaxing tendons to reduce pain.	Removing heat with damp from intestine; next relieving mild exterior syndrome.
Main Indication	Dysentery or diarrhea, with mucous and pus-bloody stools, abdominal pain with tenesmus.	Acute diarrhea with yellow, foul and watery stools, fever, aversion to wind, restlessness, thirst.

Questions for Review and Thinking

1. What are the basic manifestations of *Shaoyang* pattern? Could you explain their pathological mechanisms respectively?

2. How do you understand the pathogenesis of *Shaoyang* pattern? Why *Xiao Chaihu Tang* can be seen as its main formula?

3. Why did *Zhang Zhongjing* say, "*Chaihu Tang* syndrome, which can be confirmed according to only one main symptom"? What clinical significance does this viewpont have?

4. What are main differences between *Xiao Chaihu Tang* syndrome and *Da Chaihu Tang* syndrome in indication and pathogenesis? Why?

5. How to understand the pathogenesis and main indications of *Chaihu Guizhi Ganjiang Tang* syndrome?

6. What kind of syndrome should be treated by *Chaihu Jia Longgu Muli Tang*? How do you apply this formula clinically?

Chapter IV

Differentiation of Symptoms, Pulses and Treatment of *Taiyin* Pattern

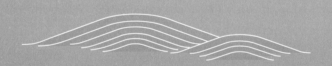

Article 273

Taiyin **pattern is characterized with abdominal fullness, vomiting, poor appetite with stagnated food in the stomach, gradually aggravating diarrhea, and sometimes abdominal pain. There would be distending-hardness in the epigastric region if catharsis is used carelessly for it.**

Synopsis	The programmatic symptoms of *Taiyin* pattern and its treatment contraindication.
Commentary	*Taiyin* pattern is the first and milder one of the three *Yin* patterns, and has a basic pathogenesis, i.e., deficiency of spleen-*Yang* leading to retention of cold-damp in the middle *Jiao*. Retention of cold-damp impedes *Qi* flow of the middle *Jiao*, so abdominal fullness and pain occur; deficiency of spleen-*Yang* denotes hypofunction of the spleen in transformation and transportation of foodstuffs, so there are poor appetite and stagnated food in the stomach; the spleen failing to ascend clear *Yang* and stomach failing to descend turbid *Yin* due to retention of cold-damp, so gradually aggravated diarrhea and vomiting occur. The above mentioned five symptoms can be seen as the major and typical manifestations of *Taiyin* pattern caused by its basic pathogenesis, and also are the key points for differentiation of this pattern.
Application	*Taiyin* pattern belongs to a deficiency-cold syndrome in the middle *Jiao* instead of the whole body, *Yang* deficiency of the spleen is primary, and cold-damp is secondary, thus pertaining to deficiency with excess syndrome. The five symptoms mentioned-above may happen partly or one symptom is severe while others are mild.

Article 277

Chronic diarrhea not caused by mistreatment and absence of thirst are ascribed to *Taiyin* pattern because of deficiency-cold in the spleen, thus should be warmed with *Sini Tang* or the like.

Synopsis	The focus on differentiation, pathogenesis and treatment of *Taiyin* pattern.

Commentary

The article emphasizes the keypoint for differentiation, pathogenesis and treatment of *Taiyin* pattern. Chronic diarrhea not caused by mistreatment suggests that the diarrhea is ascribed to deficiency of spleen-*Yang* instead of an excess or heat syndrome; meanwhile, the absence of thirst indicates either *Yang* deficiency of the spleen or cold-damp accumulation in the stomach, which differs from *Yangming* pattern, presenting thirst with desire for cold drinks, and constipation or unsmooth defecation; it differs from the *Shaoyin* pattern, marked by cold limbs and severer diarrhea with thirst. So choronic diarrhea and no thirst are regarded as two typical presentations and can reflect the pathological essence of the *Taiyin* pattern.

Aiming at the basic pathogenesis, the main therapeutic rule for *Taiyin* pattern is warming the spleen-*Yang* to dispel cold-damp in the middle *Jiao* first. For example, *Lizhong Tang* is used for its mild cases located in the middle *Jiao*, while *Sini Tang* for its severe cases happening throughout the whole body.

Application

"Be warmed with *Sini Tang* or the like" suggests that *Taiyin* pattern should be remedied by warming-tonifying; however, *Sini Tang* is a main formula for the *Shaoyin* pattern which is more serious than *Taiyin* pattern, so most TCM scholars in the later ages thought *Lizhong Tang* (or *Wan*) is more suitable for it.

Section 2   Concomitant and Transmuted Syndromes of *Taiyin* Pattern

Article 276

The *Taiyin* pattern with a floating pulse may be treated by diaphoresis, and *Guizhi Tang* is suitable.

Article 163

The *Taiyang* syndrome with unrelieved exterior symptoms but treated with catharsis several times, is then marked by incessant diarrhea accompanied with fever on the body surface, epigastric stuffiness and hardness, which indicate that the disease is in both the exterior and interior, which should then be treated mainly by *Guizhi Renshen Tang*.

Guizhi Renshen Tang	*Guizhi* 12 g, *Renshen* 9 g, *Ganjiang* 9 g, *Baizhu* 9 g and *Zhi Gancao* 12 g
Synopsis	The symptoms and treatment of *Taiyin* pattern with mild exterior syndrome after the *Taiyang* syndrome has been treated wrongly by catharsis.
Commentary	The *Taiyang* exterior syndrome treated by catharsis several times will damage *Yang Qi* of the spleen-stomach, and then lead to further retention of cold-damp pathogen in the middle *Jiao*, marked by incessant diarrhea, epigastric fullness and hardness, tastelessness in the mouth, absence of thirst, clear urine, pale tongue with white-greasy coating and a moderate-weak pulse.
	Meanwhile, the mild exterior syndrome still exists, characterized with

fever, aversion to cold and headache to a certain degree. Actually, this is an amalgamation of *Taiyang* and *Taiyin* patterns but *Taiyin* pattern is predominant to *Taiyang* one.

Guizhi Renshen Tang can be regarded as *Li Zhong Tang* plus *Guizhi. Li Zhong Tang*, also named *Renshen Tang*, is used for *Taiyin* syndrome, and *Guizhi* is added for the mild exterior syndrome. Furthermore, it also verifies that *Lizhong Tang* is just the basic formula of *Taiyin* pattern.

Application

Guizhi Renshen Tang has been applied in two aspects: *Taiyin* pattern with mild *Taiyang* syndrome, and deficiency-cold of the spleen-stomach with cold-damp retention. According to the recent clinical reports, it is often used for the treatment of chronic superficial gastritis, atrophic gastritis, gastric ulcer, duodenal bulbar ulcer, chronic colitis, and so on.

Article 279

After *Taiyang* pattern was wrongly treated by catharsis, there is abdominal fullness with occasional pain, which is similar to the *Taiyin* pattern, and it should be treated mainly by *Guizhi Jia Shaoyao Tang*; if there are severe abdominal pain with tenderness and constipation, it should be treated mainly by *Guizhi Jia Dahuang Tang*.

Guizhi Jia Shaoyao Tang

Guizhi Tang plus *Baishao* 9 g.

Guizhi Jia Dahuang Tang

Guizhi Tang plus *Baishao* 9 g and *Dahuang* 6 g.

Synopsis

The chief symptoms and treatment of two syndromes similar to that of the *Taiyin* pattern but is actually mixed syndrome of deficiency and excess.

Commentary

Taiyang pattern treated carelessly by catharsis may result in *Yang Qi* deficiency of the spleen leading to further *Qi*-blood stagnation of the gastrointestinal tract. Therefore, in this case some cold-deficiency symptoms are similar to *Taiyin* pattern, but the abdominal fullness and pain indicate an evident stagnation of *Qi* and blood in the abdomen. This isn't a simple *Taiyin* pattern, and belongs to mixed syndrome of deficiency and excess.

Since it is not a real *Taiyin* pattern, *Lizhong Tang* or *Sini Tang* can't be used. In *Guizhi Jia Shaoyao Tang,* a large dose of *Baishao* combined with *Guizhi*, *Shengjiang* and *Gancao* can warm spleen-*Yang* to propel the flow of *Qi* and blood, and relax the tendons to relieve pain. In *Guizhi Jia Dahuang Tang, Dahuang* is added to lower intestinal *Qi* and helps *Baishao* to remove blood stasis and stop pain, thus the formula is used for the syndrome with a more serious stagnation of *Qi* and blood and intestinal obstruction, marked by more serious abdominal pain with tenderness and constipation.

Application

These two formulas originated from *Guizhi Tang*, but their action in relieving exterior syndrome is weaker than *Guizhi Tang,* and their action in activating Qi-blood and unblocking intestinal *Qi* is stronger than it.

Moreover, both can't be used for *Taiyin* pattern like *Lizhong Tang*, because of their stronger action in removing blood stasis and purgation. So they may be used for treating cold, influenza, I.B.S. enteritis, urticaria and so on, only if their pathogeneses are the same as those of both formulas.

Article 280

If *Taiyin* pattern usually manifested as a feeble pulse with persistent spontaneous diarrhea needs to be treated by *Dahuang* and *Shaoyao,* giving both in a small dose, because such purgatives easily impair stomach-*Qi*, then leading to the deteriorated disorders.

Synopsis

Cautiously use purgatives and very cold natured drugs for severe *Taiyin* pattern with persistent diarrhea.

Deficiency-cold in the middle *Jiao* is a basic pathogenesis of *Taiyin* pattern, in the article "a feeble pulse with persistent spontaneous diarrhea" show that it pertains to a serious deficiency-cold syndrome, so cannot be treated by purgatives and very cold natured drugs like *Dahuang* and *Baishao*, because they can damage the spleen-stomach and weaken *Yang Qi*, thus the *Taiyin* pattern would deteriorate. Of course, some complicated cases may need to be treated by such herbal medicines as *Dahuang* and *Baishao*, for purgation, clearing heat, nourishing *Yin* or activating *Qi* and removing blood stasis; however, these drugs should be in small doses, so as to keep the herbal medicines' therapeutic functions and avoid the unfavorable actions of them.

Application
The major academic viewpoint of the article is not only suitable for *Taiyin* pattern, but also suitable for all patients featured by two opposite pathogeneses, in which the principal medicines are given in large doses and aim at the first pathogenesis, while other medicines in small doses are used for the secondary and opposite pathogenesis.

Article 259

A cold-induced disease appearing after diaphoresis, marked by yellowish skin and eyes, resulting from the accumulation of cold-damp in the interior, cannot be treated by catharsis, and should be treated by removing cold and damp in the interior.

Synopsis
The main pathogenesis, therapeutic principle and contraindication of *Yin*-jaundice.

Commentary
The improper diaphoresis used for cold-induced disease may impair *Yang Qi*, which leads to cold-damp retention in the interior, referring mainly to the spleen-stomach located in the middle *Jiao*, further resulting in an adverse flow of the bile due to *Qi* obstruction of the liver-gallbladder, and manifesting as dim-yellowish skin, eyes and urine, aversion to cold, heavy body, spiritlessness, tastelessness and greasiness in the mouth, poor appetite, nausea or vomiting, epigastric stuffiness, abdominal distention,

loose stools, pale-puffy tongue with white-thick-slippey coating, and a deep-slow or soft-moderate pulse, which can be seen as a concurmitant or transmuted syndrome of the *Taiyin* pattern, and is called as *Yin-*jaundice afterwards.

Application

The medical specialists in the later ages created some effective formulas for this syndrome, e.g., *Yinchen Wei Ling Tang*（茵陈胃苓汤）and *Yinchen Zhu Fu Tang*（茵陈术附汤）, *which* can warm *Yang* and invigorate the spleen to relieve jaundice by dispelling cold-damp, both according to the therapeutic principle of this article.

Questions for Review and Thinking

1. What are the basic manifestations of *Taiyin* pattern? Why does the pattern have such manifestations?

2. What are the main therapeutic principle and contraindicated rulese when treating *Taiyin* pattern? Why?

3. How do you understand the major pathogenesis, commonly seen symptoms and basic therapeutic principle of *Yin*-jaundice?

Chapter V

Differentiation of Symptoms, Pulses and Treatment of *Shaoyin* Pattern

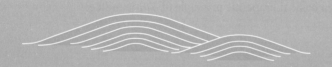

——— **Article 281** ———

Shaoyin pattern is characterized by a faint-thready pulse and drowsiness but also with sleeplessness.

Synopsis   The principal manifestations of *Shaoyin* pattern.

Commentary   Shaoyin pattern is marked mainly by severe deficiency of both *Yang* and *Yin* of the heart-kidney involving in the whole body. A faint pulse indicates exhaustion of *Yang Qi* leading to forceless circulation of blood, and a thready pulse suggests a depletion of *Yin* blood in the vessels. Drowsiness but also with sleeplessness（*Dan Yu Mei* 但欲寐）signifies a very low spiritual state and implies the common hypofunctions of essence, *Qi* and mind due to failure of the heart and kidney, since the heart dominates blood-vessels and controls mental activities, while the kidney stores vital essence and is seen as the origin of *Yin* and *Yang* of the whole body. Therefore, the two presentations can reflect the pathological feature of *Shaoyin* pattern, which is more seriously deficient than the *Taiyin* pattern. and can thus be considered as the principal manifestations in all of syndromes of the pattern.

Application   *Shaoyin* pattern in *Shanghan Lun* signifies the serious debility of the heart and kidney, represents a fundmental deficiency of *Yang* and/or *Yin* in the whole body, thus is thought of as the deepest and weakest and sometimes dangerous *Yin* pattern. The faint-thready pulse and a drowsy- sleepless mental state may appear not serious, but would really reflect the exhaustion of both *Yang* and *Yin* of the whole body, as well as depletion of the essence, *Qi* and mind, which entail the basic pathogenesis of *Shaoyin* pattern. So, the two manifestations are commonly seen in patients with this pattern no matter it is whether a cold-transformation syndrome or a heat-transformation one.

Article 282

Shaoyin pattern manifests as frequent nausea, fidgets, drowsiness with sleeplessness, chronic diarrhea for 5 or 6 days, and thirst, belonging to Shaoyin pattern, and furthermore, results from Yang deficiency leading to inability to distribute body fluid into the mouth, creating a desire to drink. If the urine is clear and copious, the Shaoyin symptoms become evident, as deficiency-cold in the lower Jiao gives rise to the failure to control urination, thus the urine is clear and copious.

Synopsis

The primary symptoms and pathogenesis of Shaoyin cold-transformation syndrome.

Commentary

Shaoyin pattern is divided into two basic syndromes, the majority of the cases is ascribed to cold-transformation syndrome（寒化证）arising from Yang deficiency of the heart and kidney, and the minority to heat-transformation syndrome（热化证）from Yin deficiency.

This article can be seen as an outline of the former. Yang deficiency leads to failure of the stomach to descend, thus with desire for vomiting: but on an empty stomach, thus nothing is vomited out, i.e., nausea. The deficient Yang floats upward, thus disturbing the mind, then fidgets happen; deficiency of both Yang and Yin of the heart and kidney brings about mental weariness, hence marked by drowsiness but also sleeplessness. The spleen-Yang fails to be warmed by kidney-Yang, so the food and drink fail to be digested and absorbed normally, thus diarrhea appears. Deficiency of the kidney-Yang also gives rise to the body fluid retaining in the interior and lacking in the middle Jiao, so thirst with desire for intake of water occurs. Protracted Yang deficiency of the kidney induces hypofunction of Qi-transformation, so there is clear and copious urine due to loosing control of urination.

Generally speaking, drowsiness with sleeplessness, chronic diarrhea, clear and copious urine, and cold limbs with intolerance of cold are the key points for differentiation of Shaoyin cold-transformation syndrome.

Application

On the basis of the article, Shaoyin cold-transformation syndrome should differ from Taiyin pattern. The former has a more serious and general

Yang deficiency of the heart and kidney, marked by drowsiness with sleeplessness, sometimes fidgets, nausea or retching (*Gan Ou* 干呕), chronic diarrhea with thirst, clear and copious urine, and a deep-thready-weak or faint pulse; the latter has a local and simple *Yang* deficiency of the spleen with mild cold-damp retention, marked with mental fatigue or sleepiness, abdominal fullness-distention, vomiting, poor appetite, chronic diarrhea with absence of thirst, and moderate-soft pulse.

Article 283

A patient presenting a tense pulse on both *Yin* and *Yang* positions, and profuse sweating, suggests *Yang* exhaustion, and belongs to *Shaoyin* pattern, in which there should be sore throat in addition to vomiting and diarrhea.

Synopsis	Main manifestations of severe *Shaoyin* cold-transformation syndrome.

Commentary   Here, *Yin* position refers to *Chi* portion of *Cunkou*, *Yang* position to *Cun* portion, with a tense pulse on *Cun* usually shows an exterior cold syndrome; however, this article does not mention any exterior symptom, and is believed to be caused by "*Yang* exhaustion", and belongs to a serious *Shaoyin* cold-transformation syndrome, thus, presenting drowsiness with sleeplessness, aversion to cold with cold limbs, severe vomiting and diarrhea, profuse sweating and sore throat resulting respectively from deficient *Yang* floating outward, disturbing the mind upward and disharmony between the heart and kidney.

Application   "*Yang* exhaustion" (*Wangyang* 亡阳) in later ages has been given a more special and definite meaning: a critically dangerous pathological state before death, caused by depletion of *Yang Qi* of a patient, manifested as an extremely cold body, massive, ceaseless, cold and thin sweats, pale complexion, feeble breathing, no thirst, a dull mind, sluggish expression, pale-moist tongue and a faint pulse that is difficult to be palpated. Obviously, the syndrome in this article is not so serious and dangerous.

Article 285

Shaoyin pattern characterized by a thready, deep and rapid pulse, belonging to interior syndrome, can not be treated with diaphoresis.

Article 286

Shaoyin pattern characterized by a faint pulse, cannot be treated with diaphoresis because it may lead to *Yang* exhaustion. A weak-unsmooth pulse indicates that *Yang* has been deficient, and cannot be treated by purgation.

Synopsis	Forbidden therapeutic rules of *Shaoyin* pattern.

Commentary	*Shaoyin* pattern, including cold-transformation and heat-transformation syndromes, belongs to a severe deficient pattern in the whole body, especially *Yang* or/and *Yin* exhaustion of the heart and kidney, thus it can be treated only by tonification instead of elimination. Diaphoresis and purgation both pertain to elimination therapies, and may consume *Qi* and body fluid, then damage *Yin* and *Yang* of the body; therefore, both are forbiden therapeutic rules.

Application	These two articles discuss the forbiden therapies of *Shaoyin* pattern in cold-induced disease, however, the principle is also suitable for all deficiency patterns in all of diseases, namely, every deficiency syndrome that cannot be treated by various elimination therapies, such as diaphoresis, emesis, purgation, warm-acupuncture and other therapies that strongly eliminate pathogens.

Article 323

The *Shaoyin* pattern with deep pulse, should be treated by urgently warming *Yang* and *Sini* Tang is appropriate.

Sini Tang	raw *Fuzi* 9~12 g, *Ganjiang* 6~9 g and *Zhi Gancao* 6 g.

Synopsis   The basic pulse, early treatment and major formula of *Shaoyin* cold-transformation syndrome.

Commentary   "*Shaoyin* pattern" here, means *Shaoyin* cold-transformation syndrome with the deficiency-cold symptoms and signs all mentioned in Article 281 and Article 282. "Deep pulse" instead of a faint-thready pulse indicates that now *Yang Qi* is going to exhaust soon, so *Sini Tang* is urgently applied for prevention of more serious syndrome, i.e., *Yang* exhaustion, implying the preventive treatment. The pathogenesis of this syndrome is due to severe deficiency of *Yang* in the heart and kidney, leading to *Yin*-cold in the interior, manifested as cold limbs with intolerance of cold, pale complexion, drowsiness with sleeplessness, diarrhea with undigested food in stool, thirst, nausea or retching, clear and copious urine, pale tongue with white-slippery coating, a deep pulse in mild cases or a faint-thready pulse.

Sini Tang is used as a basic formula of *Shaoyin* cold-transformation syndrome, because raw *Fuzi* warms kidney and heart to save *Yang* from collapse, while *Ganjiang* warms the spleen and heart to dispel cold, and *Zhi Gancao* strengthens *Qi* and harmonizes other drugs in the formula. Besides, the second and third ingredients can reduce the toxicity of the first one as well. It is called "*Sini*" because of its chief symptom, cold limbs.

Sini Tang has been considered as a representative formula for warming *Yang* to dispel cold and save one's life from collapse. It has been extensively applied to treat many severe deficiency-cold symptoms like diarrhea, vomiting, abdominal pain, syncope, vertigo, palpitation, tympanites, and edema, etc. According to modern pharmacological research and clinical reports, it possesses actions of anti-shock, raising blood presure, tonifying the heart, improving microcirculation and relieving spasm, so it can be used for different kinds of shock, myocardial infarction, hypotension, chronic enteritis, heart failure, ascites due to cirrhosis, chronic nephritis and so on.

Article 317

Shaoyin pattern marked by severe cold in the interior with false heat symptoms in the exterior, such as diarrhea with cool and thin feces mixed with indigested food, extreme cold in the limbs, and a faint pulse barely felt, but with no aversion to cold, and reddish cheeks, or abdominal pain, or retching, or sore throat, or a pulse unable to be palpated after diarrhea has ceased, should be treated mainly by *Tongmai Sini Tang*.

Tongmai Sini Tang

raw *Fuzi* 12~15 g, *Ganjiang* 9~12 g and *Zhi Gancao* 6 g.

Synopsis

The primary manifestations and treatment of the serious *Shaoyin* cold-transformation syndrome with excessive *Yin* rejecting *Yang* outward.

Commentary

The article introduces a more serious *Shaoyin* cold-transformation syndrome than *Sini Tang* syndrome with real and serious *Yin*-cold symptoms in the interior, such as diarrhea with cool and thin feces mixed with indigested food in stool, extremely cold limbs, cold sweating, or abdominal pain, and a faint pulse barely felt or no pulse palpated after diarrhea, along with some false heat symptoms externally, such as no aversion to cold, reddish cheeks or sore throat, all implying a weak *Yang-Qi* floating outward but rejected by excessive *Yin*-cold in the interior.

Tongmai Sini Tang is actually *Sini Tang* but in a double dose of raw *Fuzi* and *Ganjiang* of *Sini Tang*, so it has a stronger action of restoring *Yang* from collapse and eliminating *Yin*-cold by communicating between the interior and exterior of the body, and is effective for this syndrome, thus named "*Tongmai*" due to its strong effect to unblock vessels and restore the normal pulse.

| Application | *Tongmai Sini Tang* is usually applied for the severe cases of *Sini Tang* syndrome, marked mainly by serious cold limbs, retching, diarrhea with indigested food in stool and a faint pulse that is barely felt. According to the original record, add Congbai 24 g to communicate *Yin* and *Yang* in case of a reddish face; add *Baishao* 6 g to relax tendons in case of abdominal pain; add *Shengjiang* 6 g to lower stomach-*Qi* in case of vomiting; add *Jiegeng* 3 g to disperse lung-*Qi* for easing the throat; and add *Renshen* 6 g to reinforce *Qi* for activating blood flow in case of still no pulse palpated after diarrhea has ceased. |

Article 315

Shaoyin pattern marked by diarrhea and faint pulse, *Bai Tong Tang* should be given. If the diarrhea is incessant after taking *Bai Tong Tang*, and accompanied with more serious cold limbs, without presence of a pulse, retching and restlessness, should be treated mainly by *Bai Tong Jia Zhudanzhi Tang*. The sudden appearance of the patient's pulse indicates an impending death, but if the pulse gradually appears, this indicates an alleviation of the disease.

Bai Tong Tang	Congbai 12 g, raw *Fuzi* 9 g and *Ganjiang* 4 g.
Bai Tong Jia Zhudanzhi Tang	*Bai Tong Tang* decoction plus *Renniao*（人尿 human body' urine）40 ml and *Zhudanzhi*（猪胆汁 pig's bile）8 ml.
Synopsis	The primary manifestations, treatment and prognosis of *Shaoyin* cold-transformation syndrome with excessive *Yin* rejecting *Yang* upward, and further *Yin* depletion following *Yang* exhaustion.
Commentary	This article discusses *Shaoyin* cold-transformation syndrome with excessive

Yin rejecting *Yang* upward, known as *Yang* upward (*Daiyang* 戴阳) syndrome. In the first paragraph, there is *Sini Tang* syndrome causing severe diarrhea, reddish face and faint pulse, suggesting that an excessive *Yin*-cold rejects the deficienct *Yang* upward, so *Sini Tang* minus *Zhi Gancao* to avoid its sluggishing action, and plus *Congbai* to warm and interflow *Yang Qi* between the upper and lower body, *Fuzi* and *Ganjiang* as the main ingredients *are* still used for warming and restoring *Yang* to dispel cold-*Yin*.

In the second paragraph, there is an aggravation after taking *Bai Tong Tang* due to a strong rejection between the excessive *Yin*-cold and the *Yang*-heat, presenting as incessant diarrhea, severely cold limbs, retching, restlessness and without pulse palpated on the basis of *Bai Tong Tang* syndrome, indicating not only a more serious *Yang* deficiency with a *Qi* blockage between the lower body and upper body, but also *Yin* fluid deficiency to a certain degree arising from incessant diarrhea; thus *Bai Tong Tang* is still used for warming *Yang* to dispel cold and restoring *Qi* interflow between the lower and upper body. Especially, *Ren Niao* and *Zhudanzhi* both belonging to *Yin* fluid, are added to guide *Yang* drugs easily to enter *Yin* position of the body downward, reducing the rejection mentioned above; meanwhile, the two drugs can also complement the consumed *Yin* fluid directly to attract the upward *Yang* downward, thus relieving the *Yang* floating syndrome.

In the third paragraph, the sudden appearance of the powerful pulse after taking the decoction implies a completely revealing outward of rootless *Yang*, so having an unfavorable prognosis; while the pulse becomes gradually forceful, this denotes the rooted *Yang* restoring gradually, thus a favorable prognosis.

| Application | *Bai Tong Tang* and *Bai Tong Jia Zhudanzhi Tang* can be used respectively for serious diarrhea, vertigo, syncope, sore throat, headache, chronic infantile convulsion, child vomiting and diarrhea, and arthralgia in *Daiyang* syndrome, exclusively caused by severe deficient *Yang* upward rejected by excessive *Yin*, and severe *Yang* deficiency with mild *Yin* deficiency. Meanwhile, they are also applied for allergic shock, enterogastritis, Raynaud's disease, simple dyspepsia with dehydration, and chronic pharyngitis in Western medicine. |

Article 316

Shaoyin pattern unrelieved for 2 to 3 days or 4 to 5 days, marked by abdominal pain, dysuria, heaviness and pain of limbs, and spontaneous diarrhea, possibly with cough, clear and copious urine, severe diarrhea, or vomiting, indicate water retention in the interior, and should be treated mainly by *Zhenwu Tang*.

Zhenwu Tang	prepared *Fuzi* 9 g, *Fuling* 9 g, *Shengjiang* 9 g, *Baizhu* 6 g and *Baishao* 9 g.
Synopsis	The main symptoms and treatment of *Shaoyin* pattern with Yang decline leading to water retention.
Commentary	*Shaoyin* cold-transformation syndrome lasting for several days must entail a more serious deficiency of kidney-*Yang*, which results in water retention in the interior due to disturbance of *Qi*-transformation with dysuria. When water pathogen overflows into the skin and muscles, it manifests as heavy and painful limbs or edema; water flowing downward and obstructing *Qi* movement, leading to abdominal pain and diarrhea; water pathogen attacking upward the lung, yields cough; and water pathogen intruding into the stomach, yields vomiting.
	When weak kidney-*Yang* fails to control urination, there may be clear and copious urine and severe diarrhea. Article 82 in Chapter 1 mentions the different symptoms of *Zhenwu Tang* syndrome, but the underlying pathogenesis remains the same.
Application	The analysis on each ingredient, general actions and application of *Zhenwu Tang* can be referenced in Article 82.
	There are the following modifications of this formula in the original text of this article: add *Wuweizi* to astringe lung-*Qi* to stop cough, and add *Xixin* and *Ganjiang* to warm the lung and dispel cold water retention in case of cough; remove *Fuling* to avoid excessive urination in case of clear and copiuos urine; remove *Baishao* due to its cold-greasy nature and add *Ganjiang* due to its warming *Yang* action in case of severe diarrhea; and add *Shengjiang* up to doses of 24 g for warming the stomach and lowering *Qi* to relieve vomiting.

Article 304

Shaoyin pattern lasting for one or two days, marked by absence of thirst and aversion to cold on the back, should be treated with moxibustion and Fuzi Tang.

Article 305

Shaoyin pattern marked by generalized pain, cold limbs, painful joints and deep pulse, should be treated mainly by Fuzi Tang.

Fuzi Tang	prepared *Fuzi* 18 g, *Baizhu* 12 g, *Baishao* 9 g, *Fuling* 9 g and *Renshen* 6 g.
Synopsis	The main manifestations and treatment of *Shaoyin* pattern with cold-damp stagnation in the meridians.
Commentary	*Shaoyin* cold-transformation syndrome caused by severe deficiency of *Yang Qi* of both the heart and kidney, then easily brings on endogenous cold-damp retention in the muscles, tendons and joints as well as obstruction in the meridians and collaterals, so characterized by pain in the joints and whole body, cold limbs, aversion to cold especially on the back, absence of thirst, listlessness with sleepiness, pale-purplish tongue with white-greasy coating, and a deep-thready-tense pulse.

In *Fuzi Tang*, *Fuzi* in a large dose warms *Yang* to dispel cold-damp as a chief ingedient, *Renshen* assists *Fuzi* to strengthen the primary *Yang Qi*, *Baizhu* and *Fuling* invigorate spleen to remove damp, and *Baoshao* promotes blood circulation and relaxes the tendons to relieve pain. Consequently, it has a strong action to warm *Yang* to dispel cold-damp and relieve pain. Contrasting between *Fuzi Tang* and *Zhenwu Tang*, the former has double dose of *Fuzi* and *Baizhu* with added *Renshen,* so it has a stronger action in strengthening *Yang Qi* to relieve pain, while the latter is with added *Shengjiang* and without *Renshen,* so it has a stronger action in dispersing outward and removing the water pathogen to reduce edema.

Application   *Fuzi Tang* has been used for a lot of painful disorders, such as painful *Bi*, muscular pain, lumbago, chest pain, abdominal pain, as well as enuresis, leucorrhagia, edema, palpitation and habitual abortion, only if they are ascribed to a serious deficiency of *Yang Qi* of the heart and kidney with cold-damp retention in the exterior and meridians. Meanwhile, it is often applied at present to treat rheumatic arthritis, rheumatoid arthritis, sciatic neuralgia, coronary heart disease with angina pectoris, myocardial infarction, chronic heart failure, atrophic gastritis, chronic enteritis, nephritis, hepatitis, pelvic inflammation, Meniere's disease and prolapse of internal organs in Western Medicine.

Contrast Pathogenesis of the four Formulas to Relieve Bodily Pain

Mahuang Tang	Wind-cold exterior excess syndrome
Guizhi Xinjia Tang	Deficiency of both *Qi* and blood with mild wind-cold exterior syndrome
Guizhi Jia Fuzi Tang	*Yang* deficiency of both exterior and interior with invasion by wind-cold-damp
Fuzi Tang	*Yang* decline of the heart and kidney with cold-damp in the meridians

Article 307

Shaoyin pattern lasting for 2 or 3 days to 4 or 5 days, marked with abdominal pain, dysuria, and protracted diarrhea with purulent and bloody stools, should be treated mainly by *Taohua* Tang.

Taohua Tang   *Chishizhi* 30 g, *Ganjiang* 6 g and *Jingmi* 30 g. *Chishizhi* 15 g and other two drugs are decocted with water 500 ml, and remove the dregs after the rice has done completely, then one third decoction is taken orally with the powder of *Chishizhi* 5 g, 3 times a day. Discontinue the rest of the decoction if diarrhea has been relieved after taking the first portion of the decoction.

Main manifestations and treatment of *Shaoyin* cold-transformation syndrome marked by protracted diarrhea with purulent and bloody stools.

Shaoyin pattern with protracted diarrhea suggests a longer *Yang* deficiency of kidney and spleen. The protracted diarrhea implies gradual impairment of *Yang Qi*, which can further lead to *Qi* sinking of the spleen and injury of intestinal collaterals, thus presenting incontinence of defecation and purulent and bloody stools with a dim pale color and without foul odor.

The cold-damp accumulation in the middle *Jiao* due to *Yang* deficiency gives rise to abdominal pain, alleviated by warmth and pressure. Here, dysuria results from both hypofunction of *Qi*-transformation due to both kidney-*Yang* deficiency and inadequacy of body fluid after prolonged diarrhea.

Taohua Tang can warm *Yang* to dispel cold and stop diarrhea by astringing, because a half amount of *Chishizhi* in decoction warms the spleen to invigorate its function, another half of *Chishizhi* in powder is directly taken orally and acts on the intestinal mucosa to reduce diarrhea and bleeding by astringing; meanwhile, *Ganjiang* helps *Chishizhi* to warm *Yang* and dispel cold-damp in the middle *Jiao,* and *Jingmi,* a polished round-grained nonglutinous rice, strengthens *Qi* and complements body fluid. As the decoction becomes pink in color like peach flowers（*Taohua* 桃花）, this is due to cooked rice stained by *Chishizhi,* thus named as *Taohua Tang.*

Taohua Tang can be used for protracted diarrhea, dysentery and hematochezia only caused by *Yang* deficiency of the spleen-kidney leading to inability to control defecation regardless of either purulent-bloody stool being discharged or not.

According to recent TCM clinical reports in China, this formula is effectively applied for such diseases in Western medicine, as enteritis, ulcerative colitis, bacterial dysentery, amebic dysentery, ileotyphus, hemorrhage of upper digestive tract, functional uterine bleeding and leucorrhagia.

Article 301

Shaoyin pattern just starts, but there is fever and a deep pulse, it should be treated mainly by *Mahuang Xixin Fuzi Tang*.

Mahuang Xixin Fuzi Tang

Mahuang 6 g, prepared *Fuzi* 9 g and *Xixin* 6 g.

Article 302

Shaoyin pattern has lasted for 2 or 3 days, and should be treated by *Mahuang Fuzi Gancao Tang* to induce sweating slightly because of no obvious interior symptoms.

Mahuang Fuzi Gancao Tang

Mahuang 6 g, prepared *Fuzi* 9 g and *Zhi Gancao* 6 g.

Synopsis

The main manifestations and treatment of *Shaoyin* cold-transformation syndrome with mild exterior syndrome.

Commentary

These two articles both discuss the amalgamated syndrome of both *Taiyang* and *Shaoyin* patterns. At the beginning of *Shaoyin* cold-transformation syndrome, the *Taiyang* exterior syndrome still exists, and here, fever and a deep pulse are regarded as the representative symptoms of an mild exterior syndrome and *Shaoyin* cold-transformation syndrome respectively, while the other manifestations may have severe aversion to cold, headache, bodily pain, listlessness, lassitude, and pale tongue with white-thin-moist coating. However, the cold-transformation syndrome with the exterior syndrome is not serious, thus there are such terms as "just starts", "no obvious interior symptoms", and "induce sweating slightly" in the article.

Mahuang Fuzi Xixin Tang and *Mahuang Fuzi Gancao Tang* are both suitable for this syndrome, since *Fuzi* strengthens *Yang* to dispel cold,

Mahuang induces sweating to relieve exterior syndrome, and *Xixin* acts on both the exterior and interior, while *Gancao* supports *Qi* and slows down the actions of *Fuzi* and *Mahuang*. So the latter formula is milder than the former one.

Application

These two formulas have been used mainly for common cold, headache, *Bi* disease, lumbago, cough, asthma, lung-distention and fluid-retention, all caused by *Yang* deficiency with mild exterior syndrome or cold-damp in the meridian. They can be applied to treat many diseases in Western medicine, such as cold, chronic bronchitis, bronchial asthma, pulmonary emphysema, pulmonary heart disease, interstitial pneumonia, bradycardia, hypotension, lumbar myositis, hypertrophic arthriris, rheumatic arthritis, hyperosteogeny, sciatica, angioneurotic headache, allergic rhinitis, etc.

Article 324

The *Shaoyin* pattern with immediate vomiting just after eating, or frequent nausea with oppressive chest. At the beginning of a disease, there are cold hands and feet and a wiry-slow pulse, suggesting an excess syndrome in the chest, but it cannot be treated by catharsis, and should be treated by emesis. If there is cold fluid-retention above the diaphragm, manifested as retching, it cannot be treated by emesis and should be treated by warming, so *Sini Tang* is suitable.

Synopsis

Syndrome differentiation between *Shaoyin* cold-transformation with cold-fluid retention and shaped pathogen obstruction in the chest as well as their treatment.

Commentary

In the first paragraph "*Shaoyin* pattern" denotes a severe cold-deficiency syndrome due to *Yang* deficiency, which may lead to endogenous production of fluid-retention with *Qi* stagnation or *Qi* adverse ascending in the stomach, where there is serious vomiting, or retching or nausea. However, the second and third paragraphs belong to an excess-cold syndrome and deficiency-cold one, on the basis of inferring the pathogenesis from the pulse and treatment.

The syndrome in the second paragraph is marked by wiry-slow pulse and treated by emesis, suggesting the shaped phlegm or fluid-retention in the chest above the diaphragm has occurred; but the syndrome in the third paragraph is marked by retching and cold fluid-retention in the chest resulting from *Yang* deficiency, so treated by warming and *Sini Tang*, suggesting a severe *Shaoyin* cold-transformation syndrome.

Application

This article tells us how an excess and deficiency can be transformed from each other, thus forming a mixed syndrome of both. Moreover, an excess syndrome should be further judged by what pathogen is in which location, then the treatment may greatly differ. For example, wind-cold exterior syndrome is treated by diaphoresis and *Mahuang Tang*; a shaped pathogen stagnating in the upper *Jiao* is treated by emesis and *Guadi San*; and dryness-heat obstructing intestinal *Qi*, is treated by purgation and *Chengqi Tang*.

Article 372

A severe diarrhea with abdominal distention and general pain, should be treated first by *Sini Tang* to warm the interior, followed by *Guizhi Tang* to relieve the exterior syndrome.

Synopsis

The therapeutic principle for severe deficiency-cold syndrome with mild exterior syndrome.

Commentary

When *Taiyang* exterior syndrome is combined with the other syndrome, usually relieving exterior syndrome comes first, since the exterior syndrome happens at the beginning of the disease and belonging to *Ben*, thus treating *Ben* is priority in most cases. The interior syndrome in this case is a severe *Shaoyin* cold-transformation syndrome marked by protracted diarrhea with undigested food in stool and abdominal distention, although belonging to *Biao*, it is more serious and dangerous, so the *Biao* should be treated first, so *Sini Tang* is suitable.

Application

Zhang Zhongjing thought that exterior syndrome should be treated first in the most complicated cases, however, if the other concurrently appeared disorder is more serious and urgent, or threatening the patient's life, it should be also treated first like this article. These *Zhang*'s viewpoints fully reflect the major principles of *Biao-Ben* treatment in *Neijing*, and have influenced the formation and development of TCM therapeutics.

Section 3 — *Shaoyin* Heat-transformation Syndromes

Article 303

Shaoyin syndrome lasting more than 2 or 3 days, marked by fidgets and insomnia, should be treated mainly by *Huanglian Ejiao Tang*.

Huanglian Ejiao Tang	*Huanglian* 12 g, *Huangqin* 6 g, *Baishao* 6 g, *Ejiao* 9 g and *Jizihuang* (egg yolk) 2 pieces.
	The previous 3 drugs are decocted with 450 ml, to get 150 ml decoction and remove the dregs, then *Ejiao* is put into the hot decoction to dissolve it, and *Jizihuang* added into the warm solution and stir up it for even distribution. Finally one third is taken orally, 3 times a day.
Synopsis	The main symptoms and treatment of *Shaoyin* heat-transformation syndrome.
Commentary	*Shaoyin* heat-transformation syndrome results from *Yin* deficiency of the heart and kidney, leading to an intense fire upward and further inability of heart and kidney to exchange, presenting fidgets, failure to fall asleep, dry mouth and throat, flushed cheeks, night sweating, a feverish feeling in the palms and soles, dizziness, tinnitus or deafness, red delicate tongue with less or peeled coating, and a deep-thready-rapid pulse.

Huanglian Ejiao Tang is a basic formula used for disharmony between the heart and kidney due to kidney-*Yin* consuming and heart-fire flaming upward. In this formula, *Ejiao, Jizihuang* and *Baishao* nourish *Yin*-blood to calm the mind, *Huanglian* and *Huangqin* clear away heart-fire to relieve fidgets, so altogether have a good action to cure insomnia, fidgets and palpitation by nourishing *Yin* to suppress hyperactive *Yang*.

Application

Huanglian Ejiao Tang has been used in later ages to treat restlessness, insomnia, melancholia, palpitation, seminal emission, bleeding disorder, ulcers in the tongue and mouth, dysentery, habitual abortion, hoarseness and so on, assuming they are caused by deficiency of kidney-*Yin* with hyperactive heart-fire. In recent years, it is extensively and effectively applied for such diseases in Western medicine, such as neurosis, neurasthenia, depression, anxiety, schizophrenia, menopause syndrome, various kinds of hemorrhage, recurrent aphtha, hepatic coma due to cirrhosis, viral myocarditis, and chronic pulmonary heart disease.

Article 319

Shaoyin pattern with diarrhea for 6 or 7 days, cough, vomiting, thirst, and insomnia due to fidgets, should be treated mainly by Zhuling Tang.

Zhuling Tang

Zhuling 9 g, *Fuling* 9 g, *Zexie* 9 g, *Huashi* 9 g and *Ejiao* 9 g.

Synopsis

The main symptoms and treatment of *Shaoyin* heat-transformation syndrome with water-retention in the lower *Jiao*.

Commentary

"*Shaoyin* pattern" in this article refers to *Shaoyin* heat-transformation syndrome due to *Yin* deficiency of the heart and kidney, thus marked by fidgets, insomnia, dry mouth and throat or thirst. However, it is mixed with an obvious water retention in the interior, with the water pathogen attacking the intestine, leading to diarrhea; attacking the stomach, to cause vomiting; attacking the lung, to produce cough; and retaining in the lower *Jiao*, to cause dysuria and distending pain in the lower abdomen.

There would be red tongue with yellow-greasy coating, and a thready-rapid and wiry pulse. So in *Zhuling Tang* syndrome, water retention is first, and interior heat is second, *Yin* deficiency is mild.

This syndrome is partly similar to *Huanglian Ejiao Tang* syndrome, *ZhenWu Tang* syndrome, *Wu Ling San* syndrome and *Zhi Gancao Tang* syndrome, but they have some obvious differences in pathogenesis and manifestation, so they are unable to be confused among each other.

The ingredients, actions, indications and application of *Zhuling Tang* may be combined with Article 223 of Chapter 2 for reference.

Article 320

Shaoyin syndrome for 2 or 3 days marked by severe dry mouth and throat, should be treated by urgent purgation and *Da Chengqi Tang* is suitable.

Article 321

Shaoyin syndrome marked by diarrhea with pure bluish watery stool, epigastric pain and dry mouth, should be treated by urgent purgation, and here, *Da Chengqi Tang* is suitable.

Article 322

Shaoyin syndrome lasting for 6 or 7 days, marked by abdominal distention and constipation, should be treated by urgent purgation and *Da Chengqi Tang* is suitable.

Synopsis　　　*Shaoyin* heat-tranformation syndrome that has deteriorated into

Yangming obstruction syndrome, should be treated by urgent catharsis to preserve *Yin*-fluid.

| Commentary | These 3 articles are known as the famous three urgent purgation syndromes. Respectively, such symptoms in the articles seem mild, however, they are all seen in the later courses of *Shaoyin* heat-transformation syndrome; in other words, they are aggravated from the *Yin* deficiency of the heart and kidney, and moreover, finally forming a severe *Yangming* obstruction syndrome, i.e., extreme *Yin* deficiency and intense dryness-heat blocking in the large intestine, and the latter is more urgent and dangerous, which constitutes a vicious circle by mutual affection, which should be treated by urgent purgation and with *Da Chengqi Tang* to eliminate violent pathogens to save the exhausted *Yin* fluid. Otherwise, deterioration of *Yin* depletion and intense pathogens will lead to death. |

Consequently, here "severe dry mouth and throat" indicates *Yin* fluid exhaustion due to rampant interior heat; "diarrhea with pure bluish watery stool, epigastric pain and dry mouth" suggest the body fluid passing by the side of hard-dry stool due to intense heat in the large intestine, and *Yin* fluid is heavily consumed; and "abdominal distention and constipation" imply *Qi* blockage of the intestine due to extreme dryness-heat in the interior. Besides, the patients must have the other severe excess-heat and *Yin* exhaution symptoms, e.g., fever intensified at 3~5 o'clock pm, aversion to heat, thirst with desire for cold drinks, much sweating, restlessness, or even mania or coma with delirium, scanty-dark urine, deep red tongue with black-dry or prickled coating, and a deep-thready-slippery-rapid pulse.

These syndromes should be treated urgently with *Da Chengqi Tang* and the like, to remove the intense dryness-heat so as to preserve *Yin* first. On the contrary, *Yin* being gradually restored can reduce internal heat and promote bowel movement.

| Application | *Yang* deficiency leads to deficiency-cold syndrome, and *Yin* deficiency leads to deficiency-heat syndrome, both are seen as the common basis of *Yin-Yang* pathogenesis. However, *Yang* deficiency or *Yin* deficiency, sometimes, may be transformed into an excess-cold syndrome or an |

excess-heat syndrome, as these three articles show. Therefore, the deficiency syndrome may transform other deficiency syndromes, or may even sometimes transform excess or mixed syndromes.

According to warm disease specialists in *Qing* Dynasty, the three urgent purgation syndromes can be treated by *Da Chengqi Tang*, and also by *Xiao Chengqi Tang* combined with nourishing *Yin* or/and strengthening *Qi* drugs.

Questions for Review and Thinking

1. How do you understand the pathological essence of *Shaoyin* pattern? Why are there severe debilitated mental symptom and a pulse taken as the outline manifestations?

2. What are the main symptoms of *Shaoyin* cold-transformation syndrome? Why?

3. Try to compare among syndromes of *Sini Tang*, *Tongmai Sini Tang* and *Baitong Tang* in their pathogenesis, keypoints for differentiation and formula.

4. What are the basic differences between *Zhenwu Tang* and *Fuzi Tang* in terms of pathogenesis, indication and therapeutic principle? Why?

5. What is *Shaoyin* heat-transformation syndrome? What is its main formula? Why?

6. *Shaoyin* pattern belongs to severe deficiency syndrome, so why does it include the urgent purgation syndromes?

Chapter VI

Differentiation of Symptoms, Pulses and Treatment of *Jueyin* Pattern

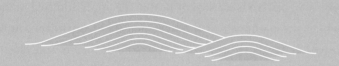

—— Article 326 ——

Jueyin pattern is marked by unceasing thirst, *Qi* rushing upward to the heart, painful and a hot feeling in the chest, easy hunger with no desire to eat, vomiting out roundworms after eating, and having an incessant diarrhea after using catharsis.

Synopsis   The outline of the major syndrome of the *Jueyin* pattern.

Commentary   *Jueyin* pattern in *Shanghan Lun* refers to a final stage of cold-induced disorders, characterized by gradually exhausted *Yin* and newly produced *Yang* simultaneously, and dysfunctions of the liver and pericardium, so there are several different complicated types of pathogeneses and syndromes in this pattern, including concurrent occurrence of cold and heat, deficiency mixed with excess, the liver pathogen attacking the spleen-stomach, and stagnation of *Qi* and blood in the body.

Consequently a mixed syndrome of both cold and heat is regarded as the major syndrome of *Jueyin* pattern. This article points out that the major syndrome of *Jueyin* pattern is marked by heat in the upper and cold in the lower, in which the pathogen of the liver possibly transformed into dryness-heat that tends to upward invade the stomach and chest, consumes body fluid and disturbs the mind, manifested as "unceasing thirst, *Qi* rushing upward to the heart, painful and a hot feeling in the chest" and "easy hunger"; when the damp-cold tends to invade the spleen and intestines downward, presenting as "no desire to eat, vomiting out roundworms after eating", abdominal pain and diarrhea.

This syndrome cannot be treated by catharsis, because purgation can further weaken *Yang Qi* of the spleen, thus causing incessant diarrhea and the other deteriorated symptoms.

The symptoms in this article can be seen as the outline of the major syndrome of *Jueyin* pattern only resulting from the lower cold and upper heat, and is only one type of the syndromes of *Jueyin* pattern. In addition to the major syndrome mentioned above, *Jueyin* pattern often involves in the disorders of vomiting, hiccup, diarrhea and cold limbs (*Jue* 厥), but some of them, don't really belong to *Jueyin* pattern, so should be differentiated from the other patterns and syndromes.

Article 338

The cold-induced disorder with a faint pulse and cold limbs for 7 or 8 days, marked by systemic cold, restlessness without temporary silence, should be Visceral Reversal Disease and not a Roundworm Reversal Disorder. The Roundworm Reversal Disorder must have vomiting out roundworms. Now the patient is quiet, then suddenly has a vexation sometimes, indicating deficiency-cold in the spleen-stomach. The vexation appears due to the roundworm going upward and passing through the diaphragm, and then silence follows for a moment. When the roundworms smell the food after eating, the vomiting and vexation occur again, thus the patient frequently vomits out roundworms. *Wumei Wan* is mainly used for Roundworm Reversal disorder, and also for prolonged diarrhea.

Wumei Wan *Wumei* 300 pieces, *Ganjiang* 30 g, Prepared *Fuzi* 18 g, *Xixin* 18 g, *Guizhi* 18 g, *Shujiao* 12 g, *Huanglian* 48 g, *Huangbai* 18 g, *Renshen* 18 g and *Danggui* 12 g.

The above 9 herbal drugs excepting *Wumei* are pounded and sieved respectively, then mixed up. Meanwhile, *Wumei* is soaked alone with vinegar over night, then remove the pips, cook 1500 g rice with *Wumei* thoroughly and put them into a mortar, next pound them with the herbal powder and honey together. Finally, process them into the pills in size of seeds of Chinese parasol, and take orally 10 to 20 pills each time before meals, and 3 times per day.

Synopsis Differentiation of Roundworm Reversal Disorder from Visceral Reversal Diseaser, and the primary symptoms and treatment of Roundworm Reversal Disorder.

Wumei Wan Syndrome can be seen as a representative type of *Jueyin* pattern, marked by mixture of cold in the lower and heat in the upper, caused by *Yang* deficiency with roundworm disturbance, known as Roundworm Reversal Disorder (*Huijue* 蛔厥). This syndrome is different from Visceral Reversal Disorder (*Zangjue* 脏厥), because the latter has an extreme depletion of *Yang Qi* in the five *Zang*-organs, characterized with serious deficiency-cold in the whole body, unceasing restlessness without temporary silencea, a dull expression, slow reaction, and a faint pulse, so this is dangerous and unfavorable in prognosis, so *Sini Jia Renshen Tang* can be used for warming *Yang* to invigorate the *Zang*-organs and strengthening *Qi* to save a life.

However, the former is milder and complicated in pathogenesis, i.e, cold in the spleen and intestines with heat in the liver and stomach, mixed with *Qi* disarrangement due to disturbance by the roundworm, thus presenting mild cold in the limbs, sometimes restlessness and vomiting out roundworms especially after eating, intermittent abdominal pain and chronic diarrhea, *Wumei Wan* can be used for it.

Wumei Wan is not only a major formula for Roundworm Reversal Disorder, but also for the lower cold and upper heat mixed syndrome of *Jueyin* pattern. Here, *Wumei* and vinegar with a sour flavor can quiet the roundworm to relieve pain; *Huanglian* and *Huangbai* with a bitter-cold nature can clear away heat in the upper body and inhibit roundworm; *Fuzi*, *Guizhi*, *Ganjiang*, *Xixin* and *Shujiao* with their pungent-heat nature can warm *Yang* to dispel cold and subdue roundworm to stop pain and diarrhea; *Renshen* and *Danggui* reinforce *Qi* and blood, and rice and honey with a sweet flavor normalize the spleen-stomch and relax tendons and muscles to relieve pain. Therefore, it has a strong action to warm *Yang* in the lower and clear heat in the upper simultaneously, next quiet the roundworm to relieve pain.

Wumei Wan has been used in later ages for abdominal pain due to roundworm, heart pain, vomiting, chronic diarrhea, dysentery, prolonged malaria, liver wind in warm disease and obstinate seminal emission only if there are severe cold and mild heat mixed with deficiency in the interior. According to recent clinical reports, it can be applied to treat a lot of diseases in Western medicine, such as intestinal ascariasis, billiary ascariasis, cholecystitis, gallstone, ulcerative colitis, bowel irritable syndrome, Meniere's disease, angioneurotic headache, leucorrhagia and pelvic inflammation.

———— Article 359 ————

The cold-induced disease originally presents with cold diarrhea, but treated by emesis and catharsis, so more serious vomiting and diarrhea happen due to mutual rejection of pathogenic cold and heat, even immediate vomiting after eating, which should be treated mainly by *Ganjiang Huangqin Huanglian Renshen Tang*.

Ganjiang Huangqin Huanglian Renshen Tang	*Ganjiang* 9 g, *Huangqin* 9 g, *Huanglian* 9 g and *Renshen* 9 g
Synopsis	The primary symptoms and treatment of *Jueyin* pattern with excess-heat in the stomach and deficiency-cold in the spleen.
Commentary	The cold-induced disease with cold-natured diarrhea indicates that *Taiyin* pattern is caused by *Yang* deficiency of the spleen-stomach, which becomes deteriorated after wrong treatment with emesis and catharsis. The excessive heat in the stomach leads to immediate vomiting after eating, thirst, bad breath, restlessness, red tip of tongue with yellow coating; while *Yang Qi* deficiency of the spleen leads to incessant diarrhea, abdominal distention and dull pain, alleviated by warmth and pressure, reduced food intake, lassitude, pale tongue with white-moist coating.

Ganjiang Huangqin Huanglian Renshen Tang is suitable for this syndrome, because *Huanglian* and *Huangqin* clear away heat in the stomach, *Ganjiang* warms the spleen to dispel cold, and *Renshen* strengthens *Qi* to invigorate the spleen, so the formula can remove the upper heat and warm the lower cold so as to relieve the rejection between cold and heat in the middle *jiao*.

By comparison, *Wumei Wan* syndrome is marked by a deficiency-cold of the spleen with milder stomach heat and roundworm disturbance, while

Ganjiang Qin Lian Renshen Tang syndrome has a more serious upper excess-heat with mild deficiency-cold of the spleen.

Application

Ganjiang Huangqin Huanglian Renshen Tang has been used for vomiting, gastric pain, dysphagia, diarrhea and dysentery due to mixture of heat and cold in the later ages, and also are effectively applied to treat peptic ulcer, chronic gastritis, gastroenteritis, dysentery, uremic gastritis and child diarrhea in autumn in Western medicine at present.

Contrast the Three Syndromes with Upper Heat and Lower Cold

Syndrome	Pathogenesis Feature	Main Symptoms
Banxia Xiexin Tang Syndrome	*Qi* stagnation due to cold and heat aggregating in the stomach with *Qi* deficiency	Epigastric stuffiness, with restlessness, fidgets, abdominal pain and diarrhea
Wumei Wan Syndrome	Severe lower cold and *Yang* deficiency with upper heat and roundworm disturbance	Cold limbs, intermittent abdominal pain,, chronic diarrhea, fidgets and vomiting out roundworms
Ganjiang Qin Lian Renshen Tang Syndrome	Severe excess-heat in the upper With mild deficiency-cold in the lower	Serious and immediate vomiting after eating, thirst, diarrhea, and abdominal pain

Section 2   Cold Syndromes of *Jueyin* Pattern

—— Article 351 ——

A patient with cold limbs and thready pulse that is almost not felt, should be treated mainly by *Danggui Sini Tang*.

Danggui Si Ni Tang	*Danggui* 9 g, *Guizhi* 9 g, *Baishao* 9 g, *Zhi Gancao* 6 g, *Dazao* 12 g, *Xixin* 9 g and Tongcao 6 g
Synopsis	The main symptoms and treatment of *Jueyin* pattern due to blood deficiency and cold coagulation in the meridians.
Commentary	This article discusses *Jueyin* pattern due to the liver blood deficiency and cold coagulation in the *Yueyin* position (the liver, pericardium and their meridians). The cold limbs result from both the cold pathogen intruding into vessels with blood coagulation, and *Yang* deficiency with failure to warm extremities; and a thready pulse almost not being felt, implies that the vessels are contracted and forceless blood circulation arises from cold coagulation and insufficient blood. According to the pathogenesis, the other symptoms may include aversion to cold, cold pain, numbness and swelling in the local extremities, head, joints, chest, abdomen and lumbar region, alleviated by warmth and aggravated by cold, or scanty or delayed menstruation, dysmenorrhea, pale complexion, bluish-purplish lips, nails and tongue with white-slippery coating.

Danggui Sini Tang can be regarded as *Guizhi Tang* minus *Shengjiang*, increasing the dose of *Dazao* and plus *Danggui*, *Xixin* and *Tongcao*. In this formula, *Danggui*, *Baishao* and *Dazao* nourish blood and promote blood circulation; *Guizhi* and *Xixin* warm meridian to dispel cold, *Baishao* and *Gancao* relax the tendons to relieve pain; and *Tongcao* activates blood flow, altogether having a strong action to nourish blood for unblocking vessels and to warm the meridian for dispelling cold; thus it can be used for *Jueyin* syndrome due to blood deficiency and cold coagulation.

| **Application** | *Danggui Sini Tang* was effectively used for a lot of painful disorders caused by blood deficiency and cold coagulation in the later ages, such as *Bi* disease, headache, chest *Bi* disease, hernia, abdominal pain, dysmenorrhea, as well as frosbite and chilblain. This formula is also extensively applied for treating some stubborn headache including migraine and cluster headache, bronchitis, heart disease with angina pectoris, myocardiac infarction, pulmonary emphysema, sciatica, koro, postoperative intestinal adhesion, Raynaud`s disease, thromboangiitis |

obliterans, periarthritis of shoulder, hypertrophic spondylitis, peripheral neuritis, pain due to cancer, postpartum bodily pain, amenorrhea, chronic pelvic inflammation, psoriasis, and frostbite of hands and feet.

Article 352

If the patient has protracted and aggregated cold in the interior, it should be treated suitably by *Danggui Sini Tang Jia Wuzhuyu Shengjiang.*

Danggui Sini Jia Wuzhuyu Shengjiang Tang	Add *Wuzhuyu* 15 g and *Shengjiang* 20 g into *Danggui Sini Tang*. The above 9 drugs are decocted with 400 ml rice wine and 400 ml water altogether, to get 350 ml decoction, then remove the dregs, and take it warmly in five times.
Synopsis	The primary symptoms and treatment of severer *Jueyin* pattern caused by intense cold coagulation in the interior and meridian with blood deficiency.
Commentary	This article introduces *Jueyin* pattern marked by a more serious cold and fluid retention in the interior, especially in the liver and stomach, characterized by severer cold limbs and aversion to cold, frequent vomiting out thin and clear spittle, obvious epigastric stuffiness and dull cold pain, and pale-bluish tongue with white-thick-slippery coating, in addition to the basic manifestations of *Danggui Sini Tang* syndrome.

Wuzhuyu and *Shengjiang* both in large doses are used for warming the *Yang* of the liver and stomach to dispel the cold and fluid retention in the middle *Jiao*, and the decoction with rice wine serves to enhance the actions of warming meridians and promoting blood circulation. This formula is different from *Sini Tang*, because it is used for *Jueyin* pattern mainly in *Xue* phase due to cold coagulation in the liver and stomach with blood deficiency, while the latter is used for *Shaoyin* pattern due to *Yang* exhaustion of the heart and kidney mainly in *Qi* phase.

Application	The clinical application of *Danggui Sini Jia Wuzhuyu Shengjiang Tang* is basically similar to that of *Danggui Sini Tang* besides having more serious indications, and it is also applied for dysmenorrhea, prolapse of uterus, progressive scleroderma, lupus erythematosus, lumbar spinal canal stenosis, etc.

Article 378

The patient with retching or vomiting out thin spittle, and headache, should be treated mainly by *Wuzhuyu Tang*.

Wuzhuyu Tang	*Wuzhuyu* 20 g, *Shengjiang* 15 g, *Renshen* 6 g and *Dazao* 9 g.
Synopsis	The main symptoms and treatment of *Jueyin* pattern due to deficiency-cold and fluid-retention in the liver and stomach.
Commentary	Retching and vomiting of thin spittle in this article are caused by the adverse ascent of turbid *Yin* (fluid-retention) resulting from *Yang* deficiency and cold coagulation in the liver and stomach, belonging to the mixture of deficiency and excess, so *Wuzhuyu Tang* is used to warm *Yang* for dispelling cold and to dissolve fluid-retention, and to normalize the stomach. Here cold pain in the head, especially in the top of head, when the cold pathogen attacks the head upwardly along the Liver Meridian of Foot-*Jueyin*. The other manifestations may include epigastric stuffiness, poor appetite, cold pain in the lateral abdomen or cold hernia, abdominal fullness, diarrhea, pale tongue with white-greasy coating, and a deep-thready-wiry pulse.

In *Wuzhuyu Tang*, *Wuzhuyu* and *Shengjiang* are both given in large doses to warm *Yang* and lower stomach *Qi* to dissolve fluid-retention and relieve vomiting; *Renshen* and *Dazao* strengthen *Qi* to invigorate the spleen, so the formula is very suitable for this syndrome.

Wuzhuyu Tang syndrome is also seen in Article 309 and 243 mentioned- |

below, and their basic pathogenesis are the same although their chief symptoms may differ, subsequently, the treatment remains the same. The explanation and application of the formula is placed after the disccusion of next two articles.

Article 309

Shaoyin **pattern marked by vomiting, diarrhea, cold limbs and extreme restlessness with a feeling of impending death, should be treated mainly by** *Wuzhuyu Tang***.**

Synopsis   Main symptoms and treatment of *Yang* deficiency in the middle *Jiao* with stagnation of turbid *Yin* (fluid-retention).

Commentary   In this syndrome, cold limbs, vomiting and diarrhea are similar to the *Shaoyin* cold-transformation syndrome treated by *Sini Tang*, but it is not really caused by *Yang* exhaustion of the heart and kidney, because extreme restlesness with a feeling of one about to die indicates that *Yang Qi* can still struggle against excessive *Yin*. This differs from severe exhaustion of *Yang* of the whole body marked by drowsiness but with sleeplessness, and intermittent and mild restlessness in the *Shaoyin* pattern. Moreover, *Wuzhuyu Tang* syndrome takes severe vomiting as the chief symptom due to adverse ascent of fluid-retention in the stomach, while *Sini Tang* syndrome takes an incessant diarrhea with undigested food in stool as the chief symptom due to serious *Yang* depletion of the kidney and spleen.

Generally speaking, *Wuzhuyu Tang* syndrome is similar to but does not belong to *Shaoyin* cold-transformation syndrome, and so is seen a doubtful syndrome of the latter, with the latter being more serious and dangerous than the former.

Article 243

Nausea or vomiting after eating belongs to *Yangming* disorder, and treated mainly by *Wuzhuyu Tang*. When the disorder worsens after taking the decoction, it belongs to a disorder in the upper *Jiao*.

| Synopsis | The pathogenesis and treatment of severe vomiting, treated by *Wuzhuyu Tang*. |

| Commentary | *Yangming* pattern belongs basically to excess-heat syndrome, but severe vomiting in this article is caused by deficiency-cold with fluid-retention in the stomach and liver according to the inference from the formula used. Therefore, the syndrome is a disorder of the stomach but does not belong to the *Yangming* pattern. The possible symptoms of the syndrome may present as nausea or vomiting out odorless and undigested food, or profuse and thin spittle, epigastric stuffiness or dull pain, poor appetite, alleviated by warmth and pressing, listlessness, lassitude, diarrhea, borborygmus, pale tongue with white-slippery coating and a deep-thready-wiry pulse, all indicating deficiency-cold of the spleen-stomach leading to production of fluid-retention and adverse ascent of stomach *Qi*. |

However, if the vomiting gets worse after taking the decoction, it suggests that the vomiting is caused by an excess heat in the lung and esophagus of the upper *Jiao*, and presents acute and sudden vomiting with foul odor, heartburn in the chest or hot pain in the epigastrium, thirst or bitter taste in the mouth, restlessness, easy hunger, upset stomach, flushed face, constipation, red tongue with yellow dry coating, and a slippery-rapid pulse.

| Application | *Wuzhuyu Tang* has a strong action to warm the liver and stomach and dissolve the cold fluid-retention in the middle *Jiao*, thus can be used for cold syndrome of the *Jueyin* pattern, and cannot be used for real *Shaoyin* and *Yangming* patterns according to the above three articles. it is not only used for vomiting, but also for stomachache, headache, vertigo, and hernia only when there is deficiency cold in the liver and stomach, or if |

Yin-turbid pathogen is attacking them or their meridians. At present, its modified formulas can be extensively applied to treat neurogenic vomiting, cardiospasm, duodenal bulbar ulcer, pyloric obstruction, nervous headache, hypertension, chronic hepatitis, epilepsy, coronary heart disease, allergic purpura, thrombopenic purpura, dysmenorrhea and muscular spasm, all having the basic pathogenesis.

Section 3 — Heat Syndromes of *Jueyin* Pattern

Article 318

***Shaoyin* pattern marked with cold limbs, or cough, or palpitation, or dysuria, or abdominal pain, or diarrhea with unsmooth feeling, should be treated mainly by *Sini San*.**

Sini San	*Chaihu* 9 g, *Baishao* 9 g, *Zhishi* 9 g and *Zhi Gancao* 9 g.
Synopsis	The primary symptoms and treatment of mild heat syndrome of *Jueyin* pattern due to liver-*Qi* stagnation with mild heat.
Commentary	Here, "*Shaoyin* pattern" doesn't mean a real *Shaoyin* pattern, but instead refers to a doubtful syndrome of *Shaoyin* cold-transformation syndrome because of its chief symptom "cold limbs", which results from *Yang Qi* failing to be distributed smoothly onto the extremities of the body due to stagnation of liver-*Qi*. The other symptoms and signs may include hypochondriac fullness and distention, oppressive chest, epigastric stuffiness and distending pain, poor appetite, or abdominal pain, unsmooth defecation, diarrhea with mild tenesmus, bitter taste in the mouth, restlessness, and a wiry pulse, all arising from liver-*Qi* stagnation and further attacking the spleen-stomach.

This syndrome can be seen as a type of *Jueyin* pattern, and differs from

Sini Tang syndrome, since this one is caused by stagnation of liver-*Qi* belonging to excess-heat syndrome, while another one caused by severe *Yang* deficiency of the heart and kidney, belonging to critical deficiency-cold syndrome.

In *Sini San, Chaihu* soothes liver-*Qi* and disperses *Yang* outward to relieve depression, *Zhishi* activates *Qi* flow to reduce stagnation, *Baishao* softens the liver by nourishing *Yin*-blood and relax the tendons to relieve pain, and finally *Gancao* harmonizes all drugs and helps *Baishao* to relax tendons for relieving pain. Importantly it has a basic action to activate *Qi* flow for soothing the liver and to disperse *Yang* outward for reducing cold limbs. Add *Wuweizi* and *Ganjiang* to invigorate the lung and astringe *Qi* in case of cough; add *Guizhi* to warm the heart-*Yang* in case of palpitation; add *Fuling* to induce diuresis for removing fluid-retention in case of dysuria; add prepared *Fuzi* to warm *Yang* for dispel cold in case of abdominal pain; And add *Xiebai* to motivate flow of *Yang Qi* in case of diarrhea with tenesmus.

Application

Sini San has an action to disperse liver-*Qi* for normalizing the stomach and to distribute *Yang* outward for propelling the flow of *Qi*-blood, so it can be seen as the first prescription to treat liver-*Qi* stagnation and disharmony between the liver and spleen, and other famous formulas such as *Xiaoyao San* and *Chaihu Shugan San* are its modifications. At present, it is extensively applied in treatment of hypertrophic gastritis, duodenal ulcer, chronic hepatitis, cholecystitis, pancreatitis, billiary ascariasis, intercostal neuralgia and costal condritis.

Contrast between *Jue* Syndromes Treated by *Sini San* and *Sini Tang*

Syndrome	*Sini San* Syndrome	*Sini Tang* Syndrome
Pathological Pattern	Depressed liver *Qi* attacking the spleen leading to Qi stagnation in the interior, regarded as a mild excess-heat.	*Yang* exhaustion of the heart-kidney leading to serious deficiency and cold in the whole body.
Main Manifestation	Slight cold limbs, or low fever, hypochondriac fullness or pain, abdominal distention, unsmooth defecation, dark tongue and wiry pulse.	Severely cold limbs with aversion to cold, abdominal cold pain, diarrhea with undigested food in stool, pale tongue and deep-weak pulse.

Article 371

Heat dysentery with tenesmus should be treated mainly by *Baitouweng Tang*.

Baitouweng Tang	*Baitouweng* 12 g, *Qinpi* 9 g, *Huanglian* 9 g and *Huangbai* 9 g
Synopsis	The main symptoms and treatment of the heat dysentery due to damp-heat in the liver invading downward into the large intestine.
Commentary	"Heat dysentery" means an acute dysentery mainly caused by accumulation of heat with damp in the large intestine leading to stagnation of *Qi* and blood, where the heat is severer than damp and deeply intrudes into the *Xue* phase and intestinal collaterals, thus marked by frequent diarrhea with mucous, purulent and bloody stools, abdominal pain with tenesmus, a hot feeling in the anus, fever, thirst, bitter taste in the mouth, restlessness, scanty-dark urine, deep red tongue with yellow-greasy coating, and a wiry-slippery-rapid pulse.
	In *Baitouweng Tang*, *Baitouweng* and *Qinpi* clear the liver heat to detoxify and cool blood to relieve bloody dysentery, *Huanglian* and *Huangbai* remove damp-heat in the large intestine to reduce diarrhea, so it is very suitable for this syndrome.
Application	*Baitouweng Tang* was often used to treat dysentery, diarrhea, hernia, leucorrhagia, reddish swelling of the eyes, characterized by heat severer than damp and intense blood heat. Nowadays, it is effectively applied for acute bacterial and amoebic dysentery, acute enteritis, trichomonal enteritis, chronic non-specific ulcerative colitis, urinary infection, gonococcal urethritis, pelvic inflammation and ventricular tachycardia in Western medicine.

Section 4 | Differentiation and Treatment of Cold Limbs

Article 337

All *Jue* disorders are caused by inability of *Yin Qi* and *Yang Qi* of the body to smoothly interflow, and here *Jue* means cold limbs.

Synopsis

The basic pathogenesis and main meaning of *Jue*.

Commentary

Jue（厥）, here, refers to a symptom, i.e. cold limbs. The symptom is not only seen in *Jueyin* pattern, but also in the other patterns in the *Shanghan Lun*. However, *Jue* in different disorders have a common pathogenesis, namely, inability of *Yin Qi* and *Yang Qi* of the human body to smoothly interflow; in another words, rejection or reverse of movement of the two kinds of *Qi,* which is caused by pathogen invasion or hypofunction of the *ZangFu*-organs.

Application

Jue（厥）in *Neijing* refers to one of two symptoms, cold limbs and fainting, or one of two diseases which are considered as their chief symptoms respectively. But in *Shanghan Lun, Jue* mainly denotes cold limbs and takeing it as a chief symptom of the disease. And according to the basic pathogenesis of *Jue* in this article, the basic therapeutic principle should be balancing between *Yin* and *Yang* of the body and promoting smooth flow of *Qi* and blood by eliminating different pathogens.

The following articles discuss different syndromes all taking cold limbs as their chief symptom, however, most of the syndromes are discussed before, thus just to mention their specific pathogenesis only.

Article 353

A patient with profuse sweating, but unrelieved fever, abdominal contractive pain, limb pain, diarrhea, cold limbs and aversion to cold, should be treated mainly by *Sini Tang*.

Synopsis The symptoms and treatment of **cold-*Jue*** disorder due to severe *Yang* exhaustion of the heart and kidney.

Article 335

The cold-induced disorder lasts for one to two or four to five days, cold limbs must be accompanied by fever, and the fever happens before the cold limbs, severe cold limbs due to equally severe fever, and mild cold limbs due to equally mild fever. The heat-*Jue* should be treated by catharsis, and reddening and ulceration in the mouth appear if it is treated wrongly by diaphoresis.

Synopsis The clinical feature and treatment of **heat-*Jue*** disorder and its therapeutic contraindication.

Article 350

The cold-induced disease marked by slippery pulse and cold limbs, indicating heat hidden in the interior, should be treated mainly with *Baihu Tang*.

Synopsis The primary manifestations and treatment of **heat-*Jue*** disorder due to excessive *Yang* rejecting *Yin* outside.

Article 355

A patient presents cold hands and feet, a suddenly tense pulse, epigastric fullness, fidgets, and hunger but inability to eat, indicating shaped pathogen stagnation in the chest, *Guadi San* is suitable for it.

Synopsis The main symptoms, pathogenesis and treatment of **phlegm-*Jue*** disorder.

Article 356

A patient has cold limbs and palpitation, should be treated by *Fuling Gacao Tang* to remove water pathogen first, then treat *Jue* disorder, otherwise, water flows into the gastrointestinal tract, leading to diarrhea.

Synopsis The main symptoms and treatment of **water-*Jue*** disorder due to water pathogen obstructing flow of *Yang Qi*.

The other *Jue* syndromes mentioned in this textbook, such as ***Qi-Jue*** (*Sini San* syndrome), **blood-*Jue*** (*Danggui Sini Tang* syndrome), **fluid retentio-*Jue*** (*Wuzhuyu Tang* syndrome), **roundworm-*Jue*** (*Wumei Wan* syndrome) and ***Zang-Jue*** (*Sini Jia Renshen Tang* syndrome), require us to read the corresponding articles for reference.

Differentiation and Treatment of Vomiting and Diarrhea

Article 377

A patient with vomiting, a weak pulse, clear and copious urine, slight fever, and difficultly cured in case of cold limbs appearing, should be treated mainly by *Sini Tang*.

Synopsis

The main manifestations and treatment of vomiting in *Shaoyin* cold-transformation syndrome.

Article 379

A patient marked by vomiting and fever, should be treated mainly by *Xiao Chaihu Tang*.

Synopsis

The main symptoms and treatment of vomiting in *Shaoyang* pattern.

The other disorders taking vomiting as a chief symptom in *Shanghan Lun* include the syndromes treated respectively by *Wuzhuyu Tang, Da Chaihu Tang, Xuanfu Daizhe Tang, Shengjiang Xiexin Tang, Huangqin Jia Banxia Shengjiang Tang, Huanglian Tang, Ganjiang Huangqin Huanglian Renshen Tang* and *Baitong Jia Zhudanzhi Tang*. So learners should make comparisons among them and master the key points for differentiation of each syndrome.

Article 370

A patient marked by watery diarrhea with undigested food in stool, sweating and cold limbs, marked by interior cold with exterior fever, should be treated by *Tongmai Sini Tang*.

Synopsis   The main symptoms and treatment of diarrhea in the *Shaoyin* cold-transformation syndrome, marked by excessive *Yin* rejecting *Yang* outward.

Article 374

Diarrhea with delirious speech indicating dry stool obstruction in the large intestine, should be treated by *Xiao Chengqi Tang*.

Synopsis   The main symptoms, pathogenesis and treatment of diarrhea in *Yangming* obstruction syndrome, arised from the water flowing downward beside heat-dry stool obstruction in the large intestine.

Article 373

A patient with diarrhea and desire for drinking, indicating heat with damp in the interior, should be treated mainly by *Baitouweng Tang*.

Synopsis   The main symptom, pathogenesis and treatment of diarrhea in *Jueyin* pattern marked by damp-heat attacking the large intestine with heat predominant to damp.

The other disorders taking diarrhea as a chief symptom in *Shanghan Lun* include the syndromes treated respectively by *Gegen Huangqin Huanglian Tang, Huangqin Tang, Lizhong Tang, Gancao Xiexin Tang, Taohua Tang, Chishizhi Yuyuliang Tang, Ganjiang Huangqin Huanglian Renshen Tang,*

Wuling San and *Wumei Wan*. So, learners should make comparisons among them and master the key points for differentiation of each syndrome.

Questions for Review and Thinking

1. How do you understand the pathogenesis and classification of the *Jueyin* pattern?

2. What main symptoms, pathogenesis and basic formula correspond to major syndrome of *Jueyin* pattern? Why?

3. Try to compare between *Danggui Sini Tang* syndrome and *Wuzhuyu Tang* syndrome in terms of pathogenesis, main symptoms and clinical application.

4. What is meaning and pathogenesis of *Jue* disorder in *Shanghan Lun*? Why can *Sini Tang*, *Sini San* and *Baihu Tang* all be used for treatment of *Jue* disorders?

5. What is basic pathogenesis of vomiting? How to distinguish between *Xiao Chaihu Tang* and *Huanglian Tang* in the application of treating vomiting?

6. What are the commonly seen pathogeneses of diarrhea? *Why Tongmai Sini Tang, Xiao Chengqi Tang* and *Gegen Qin Lian Tang* all can be used for treatment of diarrhea?

Appendixes

List of Main Reference Books

1. *Zhang Ji*, **Shanghan Lun**（伤寒论）, *Song* edition. *Bejing*: The People's Medical Publishing House, 1963

2. *Cheng Wuji*, **Annotated *Shanghan Lun***（注解伤寒论）. *Bejing*: The People's Medical Publishing House, 1963

3. *Wu Qian*, **Revised *Shanghan Lun* with annotation**（订正伤寒论注）from ***Yizong Jinjian***（医宗金鉴）. *Beijing*: The People's Medical Publishing House, 1963

4. *Li Peisheng & Cheng Zhaoren*, **Teaching Reference Book *Shanghan Lun***（教学参考书·伤寒论）. *Beijing*: The People's Medical Publishing House, second edition in 2006

5. *Xiong Manqi*, national teaching textbook: **Study on *Shanghan Lun***（伤寒学）. *Bejing*: Chinese Publisher of Traditional Chinese Medicine, second edition in 2007

Appendixes

Index of Ordinal Number of the 198 Articles

Article 1........................10

Article 2........................11

Article 3........................12

Article 4........................15

Article 5........................15

Article 6........................13

Article 7........................16

Article 11........................17

Article 12........................18

Article 13........................19

Article 14........................27

Article 15........................23

Article 16........................25

Article 16........................53

Article 17........................26

Article 18........................28

Article 20........................29

Article 24........................22

Article 26........................57

Article 28........................87

Article 29........................69

Article 31........................36

Article 32........................36

Article 33........................37

Article 34........................58

Article 35........................31

Article 36........................33

Article 38........................38

Article 39........................38

Article 40........................39

Article 41........................41

Article 43........................28

Article 44........................22

Article 46........................34

Article 47........................34

Article 53........................24

Article 54........................24

Article 55........................35

Article 58........................91

Article 59........................91

Article 61........................66

Article 62........................30

Article 63........................56

Article 64........................59

Article 66........................65

Article 67........................62

Article 69........................67

Article 71........................45

Article 73........................47

Article 74........................46

Article 76........................55

Article 82........................68

Article 83........................43

Article 84........................43

Article 85........................43

Article 86........................43

Article 87........................44

Article 88........................44

Article 89........................44

Article 90........................54

Article 91........................54

Article 93........................91

Article 94........................91

Article 95........................21

Article 96........................129

Article 97........................126

Article 99........................136

Article 100........................137

Article 101........................133

Article 102........................64

Article 103........................140

Article 106........................48

Article 107........................142

Article 112........................61

Article 118........................60

Article 124........................49

Article 125........................51

Article 134........................72

Article 135........................72

Article 137........................74

Article 138........................75

Article 146.................139
Article 147.................141
Article 149....................79
Article 151....................76
Article 152....................88
Article 154....................77
Article 155....................78
Article 156....................86
Article 157....................81
Article 158....................82
Article 159....................85
Article 161....................83
Article 163.................149
Article 165.................140
Article 166....................89
Article 168.................101
Article 169.................101
Article 170.................102
Article 172.................143
Article 173....................84
Article 176....................99
Article 177....................70
Article 180....................95
Article 181....................97
Article 182....................95
Article 183....................96
Article 185....................96
Article 186....................96
Article 189.................115
Article 194.................116
Article 199.................118
Article 204.................115
Article 205.................115
Article 206.................115
Article 207.................105
Article 210....................98
Article 211....................98
Article 212.................111
Article 213.................106

Article 214.................106
Article 215.................107
Article 219.................100
Article 220.................110
Article 223.................103
Article 228.................102
Article 229.................135
Article 230.................134
Article 236.................117
Article 237.................121
Article 238.................108
Article 239.................107
Article 241.................108
Article 242.................111
Article 243.................185
Article 247.................113
Article 248.................104
Article 249.................104
Article 252.................112
Article 253.................112
Article 254.................113
Article 255.................108
Article 257.................121
Article 259.................152
Article 260.................118
Article 261.................119
Article 262.................120
Article 263.................125
Article 264.................128
Article 265.................128
Article 266.................132
Article 267.................138
Article 273.................147
Article 276.................149
Article 277.................148
Article 279.................150
Article 280.................151
Article 281.................155
Article 282.................156

Article 283.................157
Article 285.................158
Article 286.................158
Article 301.................167
Article 302.................167
Article 303.................170
Article 304.................164
Article 305.................164
Article 307.................165
Article 309.................184
Article 315.................161
Article 316.................163
Article 317.................160
Article 318.................186
Article 319.................171
Article 320.................172
Article 321.................172
Article 322.................172
Article 323.................159
Article 324.................168
Article 326.................176
Article 335.................190
Article 337.................189
Article 338.................177
Article 350.................190
Article 351.................180
Article 352.................182
Article 353.................190
Article 355.................191
Article 356.................191
Article 359.................179
Article 370.................193
Article 371.................188
Article 372.................169
Article 373.................193
Article 374.................193
Article 377.................192
Article 378.................183
Article 379.................192

Appendixes

Index of the Formulas in this Book

(Sequenc of the 74 formulas are ranged according to order of the first letter of their Chinese phonetic alphabet)

Baihu Jia Renshen Tang 57, 58, 101, 102

Baihu Tang ....
.... 99, 100, 101, 102, 116, 136, 190, 194

Baitong Tang 174

Baitong Jia Zhudanzhi Tang 192

Baitouweng Tang 188, 193

Banxia Xiexin Tang .. 79, 80, 81, 82, 84, 85, 180

Chaihu Guizhi Tang 139

Chaihu Guizhi Ganjiang Tang 141, 142, 145

Chaihu Jia Longgu Muli Tang 142, 143, 145

Chishizhi Yuyuliang Tang 85, 86, 193

Da Chaihu Tang 140, 141, 145, 192

Da Chengqi Tang 107, 108, 109, 110, 111, 112, 113, 117, 122, 172, 173, 174

Dahuang Huanglian Xiexin Tang 77, 78

Da Qinglong Tang 38, 39, 42, 79, 93

Da Xianxiong Tang 72, 73, 74, 79, 80

Danggui Sini Tang ....
.... 20, 180, 181, 182, 183, 191, 194

Danggui Sini Jia Wuzhuyu Shengjiang Tang
.... 183

Didang Tang 49, 50, 51, 52, 121, 122

Fuling Gancao Tang 47, 48

Fuling Guizhi Baizhu Gancao Tang 62

Fuzi Tang 164, 165, 174

Fuzi Xiexin Tang 78, 79

Gancao Ganjiang Tang 69, 70

Gancao Xiexin Tang 82, 193

Ganjiang Fuzi Tang 66, 67, 93

Guadi San 89, 90, 169, 191

Gegen Huangqin Huanglian Tang 193

Gegen Jia Banxia Tang 37

Gegen Tang 36, 37

Guizhi Gancao Longgu Muli Tang 60, 61

Guizhi Gancao Tang 59, 60

Guizhi Jia Dahuang Tang 150, 151

Guizhi Jia Fuzi Tang 20, 29, 165

Guizhi Jia Gegen Tang 20, 27

Guizhi Jia Shaoyao Tang 150, 151

Guizhi Qu Gui Jia Fuling Baizhu Tang 87

Guizhi Qu Shaoyao Jia Shuqi Muli Longgu Jiuni Tang 61

Guizhi Renshen Tang 149, 150

Guizhi Tang 18, 19, 20, 21, 22, 23, 24, 25, 26, 27, 28, 29, 30, 31, 32, 33, 37, 53, 54, 56, 57, 58, 62, 69, 70, 87, 89, 90, 93, 139, 149, 150, 151, 169, 181

Houpo Shengjiang Banxia Gancao Renshen Tang..65, 66

Huanglian Ejiao Tang 170, 171, 172

Huanglian Tang 84, 85, 192, 194

Huangqin Jia Banxia Shengjiang Tang..............
....143, 192

Huangqin Tang 143, 144, 145, 193

Mahuang Fuzi Gancao Tang 167

Mahuang Lianqiao Chixiaodou Tang................
....120, 121, 123

Mahuang Tang.......... 26, 31, 32, 33, 34, 35, 36, 39, 40, 76, 165, 169

Mahuang Xingren Gancao Shigao Tang 56

Mahuang Xixin Fuzi Tang...........................167

Maziren Wan..............................113, 114, 122

Shaoyao Gancao Tang..............................69, 70

Shengjiang Xiexin Tang....................81, 83, 192

Sini San...............................186, 187, 191, 194

Sini Tang...........54, 67, 69, 148, 151, 159, 160, 161, 162, 168, 169, 174, 182, 184, 187, 190, 192, 194

Taohe Chengqi Tang....................48, 49, 50, 52

Taohua Tang................................165, 166, 193

Tiaowei Chengqi Tang.......................................
.................................91, 92, 104, 105, 109, 122

Tongmai Sini Tang 160, 161, 174, 193, 194

Wu Ling San 45, 46, 47, 48, 86, 87, 172

Wumei Wan... 79, 177, 178, 179, 180, 191, 194

Wuzhuyu Tang.....183, 184, 185, 191, 192, 194

Xiao Chaihu Tang.......126, 127, 129, 131, 132, 133, 134, 135, 136, 137, 138, 139, 140, 141, 142, 143, 145, 192, 194

Xiao Chengqi Tang..........69, 70, 106, 107, 109, 114, 122, 141, 174, 193, 194

Xiao Jianzhong Tang 20, 60, 64, 65, 93, 137

Xiao Qinglong Tang 39, 40, 41, 42, 93

Xiao Xianxiong Tang......................................75

Xuanfu Daizhe Tang 83, 84, 93, 192

Yinchenhao Tang..........117, 118, 119, 120, 123

Zhenwu Tang 68, 69, 93, 163, 164, 174

Zhi Gancao Tang.................60, 70, 71, 93, 172

Zhizi Chi Tang 55, 56, 102

Zhizi Gancao Chi Tang 55

Zhizi Shengjiang Chi Tang 55

Zhuling Tang.......................103, 104, 171, 172

图书在版编目（CIP）数据

伤寒论选读＝Selected Readings from Shanghan Lun：英文 / 成肇智，陈家旭编译.
－－ 北京：人民卫生出版社，2017
ISBN 978-7-117-25554-7

Ⅰ.①伤… Ⅱ.①成… ②陈… Ⅲ.①伤寒论－医学院校－教材 Ⅳ.①R222.2

中国版本图书馆 CIP 数据核字（2017）第 285278 号

人卫智网 www.ipmph.com 医学教育、学术、考试、健康，购书智慧智能综合服务平台

人卫官网 www.pmph.com 人卫官方资讯发布平台

Selected Readings from *Shanghan Lun* 伤寒论选读（英文）

编 译	成肇智 陈家旭
策划编辑	饶红梅
责任编辑	饶红梅
整体设计	尹 岩 白亚萍 水长流
出版发行	人民卫生出版社（中继线 010-59780011）
地 址	北京市朝阳区潘家园南里 19 号
邮 编	100021
E - mail	pmph @ pmph.com
购书热线	010-59787592 010-59787584 010-65264830

印 刷	北京顶佳世纪印刷有限公司
经 销	新华书店
开 本	787×1092 1/16 印张：14
字 数	323 千字
版 次	2017 年 12 月第 1 版 2017 年 12 月第 1 版第 1 次印刷
标准书号	ISBN 978-7-117-25554-7/R·25555
定 价	236.00 元